D1558650

HORSES IN HEALTH AND DISEASE

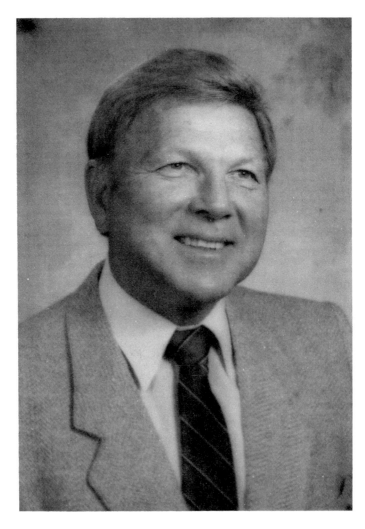

James L. Naviaux, D.V.M.

HORSES IN HEALTH
AND DISEASE

JAMES L. NAVIAUX, D.V.M.

SECOND EDITION

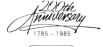

LEA & FEBIGER   1985   PHILADELPHIA

Lea & Febiger
600 Washington Square
Philadelphia, Pennsylvania 19106-4198
U.S.A.
(215) 922-1330

Library of Congress Cataloging in Publication Data

Naviaux, James L.
  Horses in health and disease.

  Bibliography: p.
  Includes index.
  1. Horses. 2. Horses—Diseases. I. Title.
SF285.3.N38   1984   636.1   84-7179
ISBN 0-8121-0935-X

PRINTED IN THE UNITED STATES OF AMERICA

Print No. 3 2 1

DEDICATED TO

My wife, Ann, my love, my sunshine
For the constant happiness you bestow upon me.
My sky without a cloud.

My four boys, Bob, Dave, Bill, and Jeff
You have given me such pleasant memories and such joys,
And of all of you I'm so proud.

And to Rena, our half-Arabian mare,
For all the patience and inspiration you have given me,
And for always being there.
Now and Always in Memory of Rena,
Who has gone to greener pastures at
The age of 27, taken with her
An unending love.

PREFACE

The purpose of my writing this book was to help the inexperienced horseman, student, and lover of horses to become more familiar with the routine needs and problems of the horse. If the reader is so fortunate as to own one, he will be more able to enjoy and care for his or her horse in good health.

The writing of this book has been a labor of love and has taken untold hours in the field and at my desk over a number of years. The results in terms of personal gratitude and appreciation expressed by so many horse enthusiasts have made the effort more than worthwhile.

The main objective in the style of writing was to, hopefully, turn unnecessarily complicated material into information that is easily obtainable, understandable, and useful. I purposely avoided using technical medical terminology, trying to write the information in an organized textbook manner and lightening the material here and there with some personal comments. I made no attempt to describe every malady of the equine species, but instead limited the discussion to the most common conditions observed by a practicing veterinarian.

I hope that this book fulfills some of your desires to know more about the care and health of the horse and that you too can experience the love and enjoyment that I have found from my association with this most noble creature of God's creation.

Walnut Creek, California   James L. Naviaux, D.V.M.

CONTENTS

PART IV—APPENDICES

PART

I

General Considerations

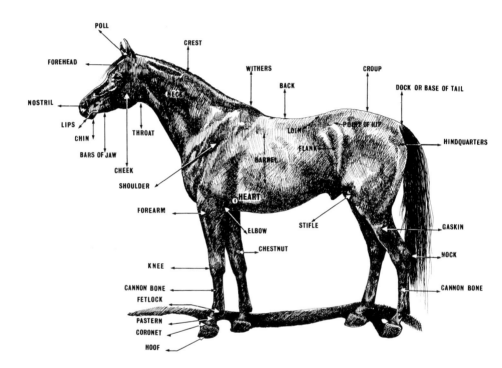

FIG. 1.   Points of the horse. (Drawing by Jeannine Quilici.)

1

The Horse

Classification: Kingdom—Animal; Phylum—Chordata; Class—Mammalia; Order—Perissodactyla; Family—Equidue; Genus and Species—Equus caballus.

HISTORY

The Early Horse

The horse has evolved to its present form over a period of 58 million years. The early Eohippus "dawn-horse" was a multi-toed animal only 12 to 14 inches high that lived in swamps. As it began to adapt to forests and prairies, it became larger and developed a large lung capacity and the single toe, which gave him speed and ability to go farther and farther from water. It has been this ability to run fast from danger that has been directly responsible for the horse's survival over such a long period of time.

Scientists believe that the earliest ancestors of the horse originated in North America and Europe, but evolution in the eastern hemisphere ended in early extinction. Thus the evolution of the modern horse took place in the Americas, as has been shown by fossil remains. By the Ice Age, about a million years ago, the horse had evolved to its present size and shape and had migrated to every continent except Australia. It is believed that at about this time the horse became extinct in North and South America for unknown reasons. It was not until the 1500s that the horse was re-introduced into this part of the world by the Spanish. The wild horses, or mustangs, in the western United States are descendants

3

of the horses that escaped from the early Spanish explorers and settlers.

The exact origin of the modern breeds of horses is not known, but three ancestral groups are considered the antecedants of present-day horses: the *Libyan* (North Africa), the *Arabian* (Arabia), and the *Flemish* horse (Central Europe). The fine-boned "hot blooded" horses of today are descended from the Libyan and Arabian breeds, and the heavier "cold blooded" draft horses are descended from the Flemish breed, which also gave rise to the Celtic pony (Ireland), from which our modern ponies are derived.

Man and the Horse

Early man most likely hunted the horse for food. The domestication of the horse, as with all of our other domestic animals, occurred in prehistoric times. The history of early man's relationship to the horse has been left to us by carvings and pictures on walls of caves. By such findings in Southwest Asia, drawings show that man was riding horseback more than 5000 years ago. It is known that the Assyrians hunted with horses about 800 B.C. The Persians, who were accomplished horsemen, used horses for hunting, sports, and war.

Horse-drawn chariots were used in Greece 1000 years B.C. Racing of "riding horses" was instituted in the Olympic games in 648 B.C. The Greeks' interest in and respect for horses are shown in their belief that their Sun God, Apollo, drove a chariot drawn by four horses across the sky each day. Their belief in Pegasus the flying horse was also testimony to their appreciation of this marvelous animal. Many early Greek coins (before 300 B.C.) had a horse or a chariot drawn by horses engraved on them.

The Macedonians were the first to fully develop the use of the horse for warfare. From these times until the first world war, the horse cavalry played an important part in all armies. Draft breeds were developed to carry knights and warriors with heavy armor. After gun powder came into use during the 1300s, lighter, faster horses were sought to replace the draft breeds. One result of this change in military attitudes is our modern light horse breeds. It is believed that the Normans in England were the first to plow with horses instead of oxen. The use of the horse also had a great influence on the recent history of North American Indians and the settling of the western United States.

The Horse Industry in the United States Today

It has been estimated that there are approximately 8.4 million horses in the United States (1983) and some 3.2 million horse owners. About 80% of these horses are owned for other than professional use. Historically, the horse population was on the increase up to 1915, at which time there was a record number of 21,431,000, almost 3 times that of the horse population today. Then it started to decline. On the other hand, mules continued to increase in population until 1925, at which time they numbered 5,918,000. Horses hit the lowest population level in recent times in 1960, when the total population of both mules and horses totaled 3,089,000. By the year 1968, the horse population was up to 6,675,000. Between 1960 and 1982, the number of registered foals had increased from 72,853 to 310,178.

Increases in Horse Populations from 1971 to 1983 in the Ten States with the Most Horses.			
	1971 USDA Estimate	1983 AHC Estimate	% Increase
1. California	406,000	850,000	52
2. Texas	625,000	780,000	20
3. Oklahoma	230,000	300,000	23
4. Montana	250,000	250,000	0
5. Ohio	205,000	248,000	17
6. Missouri	188,000	242,000	17
7. Michigan	169,000	222,000	24
8. Kentucky	170,000	220,000	22
9. Colorado	125,000	219,000	43
10. Tennessee	180,000	219,000	18

Today, there are over 150 newspapers and magazines that deal specifically with horses.

Horse owners spend $7.9 billion annually on feed, equipment, drugs, services, and related items. Over $8.3 billion is invested in horses and related assets; $2 billion is invested in land and buildings. There are more than 200,000 breeders of registered horses; more than 7300 nationally sanctioned horse shows are conducted annually. Equine events drew approximately 110 million spectators in 1975. Horses consume more than 2 million tons of formula horse feeds and 4 million tons of hay each year. Horse racing has been the number-one spectator sport for over 30 consecutive years, attracting some 77 million people annually. During 1982–83, exports of horses exceeded imports by $149 million.

Though the growth of the horse population has been on a steady upward trend for more than 30 years, many cities are experiencing some changes, with previous pastures and riding areas being turned into locations for condominiums and private homes. Also, the costs of feeding and related costs of owning a horse have sky rocketed, which is drastically affecting the number of backyard horse owners.

CHARACTERISTICS OF THE HORSE

Colors

As we know, horses come in different colors and with different amounts of white on their bodies. This fact probably gave some basis for the old reference to "a horse of a different color." The following are common horse body colors:

1. *Bay*—The body color of bay horses varies from a light tan to brown to a dark rich mahogany (blood bay). The bay horse has a black mane and tail and usually has black on the legs.
2. *Black*—A black horse should be completely black, including the muzzle and flank area. (Sun bleaching of the hair, which is usually caused by vitamin-A deficiency, should not keep one from recognizing a black coat. Black horses are not too common and are rare in the Arabian breed.)
3. *Brown*—A brown horse often appears to be black, but has brown hairs on the muzzle and flanks. (It is a relatively uncommon coat color, but is most common in the Thoroughbred breed.)
4. *Chestnut* (Sorrel)—Chestnut horses are colored in shades of red with the mane and tail usually the same color as the body. The coat may be a medium golden (light chestnut), reddish (sorrel), or deep dark red (liver chestnut). The term "sorrel" is another description used for chestnut horses, but in the western states is commonly used in reference to the more reddish chestnut. The manes and tails are sometimes silver and are called "flaxen" manes and tails. Chestnut horses never have black manes and tails. (Chestnut, bay, and gray are the most common colors among all solid-colored horses. Chestnut is the most common color of all.)
5. *Gray*—Gray is a common color among many breeds, especially in Arabians and Lippizans. Such horses have black skin. All horses that eventually turn gray are born black, but show evidence of changing when they begin to shed their baby coats at 2 to 3 months of age. Gray horses tend to get lighter with age. Many young horses, when in good general health, develop a glossy gray coat with contrasting darker blotchy areas, which is called a "dapple-gray." Gray horses with reddish overtones are called "Rose Grays." A dark gray horse with multiple small patches of whitish hair over the body is referred to as a "flea bitten" gray.
6. *White*—White horses are born with a white coat and are white throughout their lives. The skin is pink and the eyes are brown or, occasionally, blue. Many white horses are referred to as "albinos," but are not true Albinos. A true Albino has

no pigmentation on its body and has pink eyes. True albinoism in horses is not a recognized phenomenon, and if it were, it would be (as with other animals) a genetic mishap or mutant.

7. *Palamino*—The palamino color is a golden color with shades varying from light to deep gold. Palamino horses have silver manes and tails.

8. *Buckskin*—A buckskin horse has a yellowish-tan color over its entire body except for a black mane and tail and a black line running down its back.

9. *Dun*—The dun horse frequently appears to have the same coloration as a buckskin, but has the same color mane and tail as the rest of its body rather than the black mane, tail, and spinal line of the buckskin. These horses often have a slightly darker yellowish strip down their backs, but it is not always evident.

10. *Roan*—Roan horses have an intermingling of white hairs with red or black hairs. The combination of white and black gives the horse a bluish color (a Blue Roan). Horses with a combination of white and red hairs are called Strawberry Roans.

11. *Appaloosa*—Appaloosa horses have many variations and combinations of coat patterns with colorful spots. A horse that has a solid coat color over its head and body forward of its middle back and multiple spots over white hindquarters is referred to as a "blanketed Appaloosa." Many horses have a uniform base white coat with multiple spots over the entire body; these are called "leopard Appaloosas." Blotchy white skin (mottling) around the mouth, rectal, and genital areas is characteristic of appaloosas, as are striped hooves. Some foals are born a solid color and turn appaloosa by the time they are 12 to 18 months of age. The Appaloosa's color has a tendency to fade to a lighter shade with age.

12. *Pinto*—The pinto coat has large irregular areas of white and any other color. The Spanish word *pinto* means "painted," and these horses are often referred to as "Paints." The other body color is often black, brown, or palamino.

13. *Grulla*—This is a relatively rare coat color consisting of uniformly mousy gray hair over the entire body. (It is most often seen in the Quarter Horse breed.)

Markings

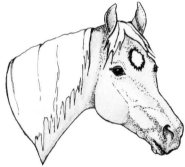

Head

Star—Any white marking on the forehead. It may be described as large, small, irregular, or faint.

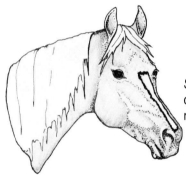

Strip—A narrow white strip, usually down the center of the face from about the level of the eyes to the nostrils.

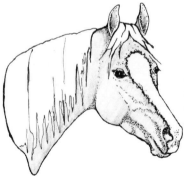

Blaze—A broad white marking down the face, usually involving the whole width of the nasal bones down to the nostrils. Blazes are often irregular and off center.

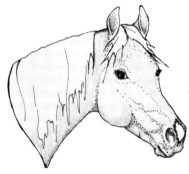

Snip—A white marking between the nostrils.

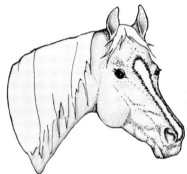

Star, Strip, and Snip—Includes all three. Basically, it appears to be a very narrow blaze.

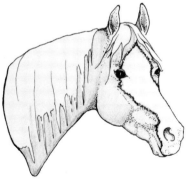

Bald Face—The face is white from the forehead to the muzzle, including one or both eyes. The eye included often has a lack of pigment in the iris and is referred to as a "glass eye." This condition does not affect the vision of the horse.

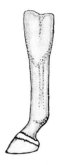

Leg

Coronet—A white strip around the coronet, which is just above the hoof.

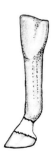

Pastern—The white extends from the coronet to just below the fetlock joint.

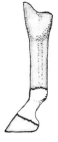

Ankle—The white extends from the coronet up to just above the fetlock joint.

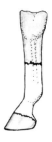

Sock—The white extends from the coronet to the middle of the cannon bone.

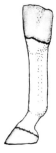

Stocking—The white extends from the coronet up to or including the knee or hock.

MODERN BREEDS OF HORSES

Arabians

Of all the horse breeds of the world, the Arabian is considered not only the oldest breed, but also the most beautiful. Modern blood lines seem to go back to 100–600 A.D., when their distinctive characteristics were established in Arabia.

Characteristics

Height—14 hands 2 inches to 15 hands 2 inches. Colors—chestnut, bay, gray, or brown (markings are common). Weight—850–1000 pounds.

Appearance

Head—small concave "dished-face" with profile that tapers to a small chiseled muzzle. Eyes—very large, circular, widely spaced, and placed low in the skull. Nostrils—large and flexible. Jaw—very deep and wide. Ears—small and characteristically curved with tips pointed inward. Chest–broad. Body—short with flat topline over croup, high tail-set, and "gay" tail carriage; the tail often curves over the horse's back when it is trotting with a floating gait. Arabians are well known for their endurance and "easy keeping" (requiring little feed) qualities. Most Arabians like people and like to be around them.

Use

Arabians are mostly used for general pleasure riding, shows, and trail and endurance rides. They are commonly used for both western and English pleasure riding, jumping, and some racing.

Thoroughbreds

The Thoroughbred racehorse is the best known of all British breeds. Its origin dates back to the 17th century.

Characteristics

Overall body refinement is characteristic. Height—15 hands 2 inches to 17 hands. Weight—1000–1300 pounds. Colors—chestnut, bay, brown, black, gray, and roan (white markings are common).

Appearance

Head—refined. Neck—slightly arched and elegant. Withers—pronounced. Shoulders—very sloping. Legs—with refined bones and long pasterns. Thoroughbreds are best known for their running ability, but are not known as "easy keepers."

Use

Thoroughbred horse racing is extremely important and popular in many countries throughout the world. In the United States, it is the number-one spectator sport in the country, drawing twice as many fans as does its next closest competition, professional football. The Thoroughbred is also extensively used for English pleasure, jumping, hunting, dressage, polo, and steeple-chasing, though there is growing concern about the abuse of two-year-old racing and steeple-chasing horses. Along with Arabians, the Thoroughbreds, deservingly, continually sell for high prices.

American Saddle Horse

The American Saddle Horse was developed in Kentucky, Tennessee, Virginia, and West Virginia, where a horse was desired with easy ambling gaits to ride over plantations and for long journies. This was mostly done between 1840 and 1890 using background bloodlines from Thoroughbreds and foundation animals of the Morgan and Standardbred breeds. Also of great influence on the breed's beginning was a Canadian horse known as the Canadian Pacer.

Characteristics

Height—15 to 16 hands. Color—chestnut, bay, brown, black, gray, or golden; Weight—1000–1200 pounds.

Appearance

Head—an alert carriage. Neck—long and graceful. Back—short and rounded with a level croup and high tail-set. It is known as a spirited animal.

Use

The American Saddle Horse is now used almost exclusively as a three- or five-gaited horse for pleasure riding or showing. It gives an easy ride with great style and animation. A park hack may be three-gaited (walk, trot, canter) or five-gaited (plus the rack and a slow gait-running walk, fox trot or slow pace). It is frequently shown under fine harness as well as under flat saddle, thus making it an excellent combination horse.

Standardbred

This is the official name of the famous American trotting and pacing horse that was originally bred in the Eastern United States as a road horse. The breed was developed from the Thoroughbred, Hackney, Arabian, Morgan, and certain pacers of mixed breeding and blood lines. This occurred mostly between 1800 and 1875. The name "Standardbred" came from the original requirement for registration, beginning in 1879, that the horse be able to trot the mile at 2:30 or pace the same distance at 2:25. This is no longer a requirement for registration. Today the animal need only be an offspring of a registered sire and dam.

Characteristics

Height—15 to 16 hands. Colors—bay, chestnut, brown, and black are most common, but gray, roan, and dun are found. Weight—850–1200 pounds, usually between 900 and 1000 pounds if it is a racehorse.

Appearance

In the main, the Standardbred is smaller, longer bodied, heavier limbed, and possesses less refinement than the Thoroughbred, but usually has good endurance, often racing mile after mile at top speed.

Use

Though the Standardbred is mostly used for harness racing, it is commonly used as a pleasure saddle horse and jumper and is often exhibited in light harness at horse shows.

Tennessee Walking Horse

The Tennessee Walking Horse was developed into a modern American breed of horses in the middle basin of Tennessee—mostly between 1890 to 1935. Also known as the "Plantation Walking Horse," it has been selectively bred for its unusual natural floating or smooth running walk that made it such a pleasure to ride over Southern estates. It was also used in early days as a work horse in the fields. Its foundation blood lines seem to include the Thoroughbred, Standardbred, Morgan, American Saddle Horse, and other native stock.

Characteristics

Height—15 to 16 hands. Colors—bay, chestnut, black, brown, roan, gray, white, and golden (white markings are common). Weight—1000–1200 pounds.

Appearance

When compared to the American Saddle Horse, the Tennessee Walking Horse is larger, stouter, and more rugged. It has a plainer head, shorter neck, lower head carriage, and is overall less elegant though more docile than the American Saddle Horse.

Use

The Tennessee Walking Horse is commonly used for pleasure riding, but is frequently seen in the show ring demonstrating its three natural gaits—the flat-foot walk, the running walk, and the canter, with particular emphasis on the running walk, which is simply an accelerated flat-foot walk with diagonally opposed foot movements. As the gait is speeded up, the hind feet usually overstep the front tracks by up to 18 inches. This movement results in a gliding "riding on a cloud" smooth gait, which has given rise to the phrase, "Ride one today and you'll own one tomorrow."

◦ American Quarter Horse

This is a breed of horse that was developed by early colonists in Virginia because of their interest in horse racing. Because no large tracks were available, they cut out "race paths" in the wilderness areas that were usually a quarter of a mile long. Thus, the horse that they bred for these tracks was called "the Quarter Horse." Interest in racing this horse spread to Maryland and the Carolinas and then to other colonies. As the West became more settled and the cattle industry grew, this horse, which was very strong, well muscled, and quick on its feet, became very popular mounts for cowboys, especially in Texas. With time and further development of the West, the popularity of the American Quarter Horse also spread and has continued to do so to the present day. Though early blood lines were of native mares of Spanish background without Thoroughbred influence in the 1760s, Thoroughbred breeding was introduced and greatly added to the horse's ability to start quickly and to its powerful muscling of the hind quarters. The official American Quarter Horse registry began in 1940.

Characteristics

Height—14 hands 2 inches to 15 hands 2 inches. Colors—chestnut, bay, and dun are the most common, but palamino, black, brown, roan, gray, and grulla also occur. Weight—1000–1250 pounds.

Appearance

There are two distinct types of American Quarter Horses. The *classic stout* is an overall well-muscled horse of a "bull-dog" type with a broad chest, large forearm, and well-developed neck, back, and powerful hindquarters. Head—with relatively small alert ears, and heavily muscled cheeks and jaw. This type is most commonly used as a stock and rodeo horse and for western pleasure riding. The more refined, usually taller *Thoroughbred type* is a "racing Quarter Horse." These horses frequently have heavy Thoroughbred lineage in their pedigrees, which has contributed greatly to the higher speeds being attained by modern Quarter Horses. Many of these horses are not only raced, but are also used for jumping and English riding activities. In general, the American Quarter Horse does enjoy an overall reputation of being an animal with a good, sensible, calm disposition, but as with all breeds and generalizations, there are exceptions.

Morgan

This American breed of light horse stems from the breeding of one little bay stallion, "Justin Morgan," which was foaled in 1793 in the Green Mountain country of Vermont. Little is known of the origin of this horse except that his ancestry must have been mainly Thoroughbred or Arabian.

By a lucky chance, his owner, Thomas Justin Morgan, was impressed by the stallion's looks, decided to try him at stud, and the results were striking. Although he was bred to ordinary mares, he produced almost exact replicas of himself. His fame spread and he was eventually purchased by the U.S. Army for a large sum of money and stood at stud in Woodstock, Vermont. He lived 32 years. Besides being the foundation stallion for the Morgan breed, he also contributed to the background of other developing American breeds, such as the Standardbred, American Saddle Horse, and Tennessee Walking Horse.

Characteristics

Height—14 hands 2 inches to 16 hands. Weight—800–1200 pounds. Colors—bay, chestnut, black, and brown (extensive white markings are uncommon). The Morgan has a compact, solidly built body with muscular, powerful shoulders and a thick neck and crest. The mane and tail are normally thick. It is known for its style, easy keeping, sturdiness, and endurance.

Use

The Morgan is most commonly used for general pleasure riding and stock work, but is considered a very versatile horse.

Hackney Horse and Pony

The Hackney breed is a heavy harness or carriage horse that originated in Norfolk and adjoining counties on the eastern coast of England. In the first half of the 18th century in the United States, a trotting-type horse that was fast and would go a distance was developed and known as the Norfolk Trotter. It was this native stock with Thoroughbred infusion from which the Hackney was later derived. Also in its lineage is the immortal Darley Arabian. In the 18th century, British hackney coaches were developed and the Hackney became specially trained for driving. The very name Hackney, and its derivative "Hack," is suggestive of the type of job the breed was to perform.

Characteristics

Height—12 hands to 16 hands. The small Hackney pony stands under 14 hands 2 inches and is registered in the same stud book. Weight—600–1200 pounds. Colors—chestnut, bay, and brown are the most common colors, although roans and blacks are seen (white markings are common and considered desirable).

Appearance

It is relatively short legged and heavy in proportion to its height. Its form is curved, with symmetry and balance, and it holds its head in an alert manner. Natural high-stepping action is probably its most distinguishing feature.

Use

The Hackney is an excellent driving animal. The Hackney horse is almost exclusively confined to the show ring today. Many Hackney ponies are used as "English mounts" by young equestrians. Many hunters and jumpers are half-bred Hackneys, and were bred to their desired size from this breed.

Appaloosa

These "spotted horses" seem to trace their early existence back some 2400 years to central Asia. They were considered sacred in Persia and were the heavenly horses of Emperor Wu Ti in China. The modern American Appaloosa horses were introduced by the early Spanish explorers, which is true of all modern horses in the western hemisphere. It seems that these horses became very prized by the Nez Perce Indians in Idaho, Washington, and Oregon around the 1730s; they were selectively bred and developed to significant numbers. The name "Appaloosa" seems to have developed after some of these horses lived by the Palouse Stream in Idaho and were called "Palouse" horses. An individual then became "a Palouse," which was passed down to become "an Appalousa." After the Indian wars in the late 1870s, many of these horses were scattered throughout the west. The Appaloosa Horse Club registry began in 1938.

Characteristics

Height—14 hands 2 inches to 16 hands. Weight—900–1200 pounds. Color—many variations, with patterns of spotting, speckling, and mottling on various background colors. A horse with spots over the loin and hips is called "blanketed;" a horse with uniform spotting over the entire body is referred to as a "leopard." An Appaloosa horse also has its eyes encircled by white; its skin is mottled, especially around the muzzle and genital area; and its hooves are vertically striped in black and white.

Appearance

The breed is recognized by the pattern of its coloration. Individuals vary greatly in general conformation. Much effort is currently being devoted to developing more refined and attractive heads in the breed; certain breeding programs are also directed toward breeding faster horses for racing.

Uses

The Appaloosa is widely used for general pleasure riding, parade, stock, and racing.

Pinto

The first Pinto horse, which is a color breed, was brought to America by the Spanish conquistadores in the 1530s. They were very popular among the plains Indians and became known as "Indian Ponies." They played an important part in affecting the life styles of these Indians, allowing them to become more effective buffalo hunters and warriors.

Characteristics

Height—14 hands 1 inch to 16 hands 2 inches. Weight—750–1300 pounds. Color—variable; it is preferred that the coat be half colored and half white, with the many patches of color all over the body, being separated by white. The most common color combinations are black and white, brown and white, red and white, and palamino and white. Two distinct pattern markings are recognized: overo, in which the white areas extend upward from the belly; and tobiana, in which the white areas extend downward from the back.

Appearance

Most Pintos are bred to have a general refined pleasure-horse appearance that falls somewhere between the tall smooth muscling of the Thoroughbred and the bulky musculature of the Quarter Horse.

Use

The Pinto is used for general pleasure riding, both Western and English styles, and shows. It is especially popular as a parade horse.

COMMON MODERN DAY PONIES

Generally speaking, any horse under 14 hands 2 inches is classified as a pony. The lack in size alone does not constitute a pony type. There are three distinct types of ponies, which are miniatures of the draft horse, the heavy harness horse, and the saddle horse. Each has its special uses.

Shetland Pony

The Shetland pony came from the Shetland Islands, which are located about 200 miles north of Scotland. The islands have a rough and rocky terrain and inclement weather most of the time. This environment has produced a rugged little pony that is a very "easy keeper." The ancestry of this present-day pony is uncertain, but it is thought to have come from a small pony stock that was found in the adjacent countries of Iceland, Scandinavia, Ireland, and Wales.

Characteristics

In many ways the Shetland resembles a draft horse in miniature, but much refinement is seen in many of the blood lines today. Height—9 hands to 11 hands 2 inches. Colors—bay, black, brown, chestnut, gray, roan, and spotted (both piebald and skewband). Weight—300 to 400 pounds. The "old time" Shetland has a somewhat plain head and neck and an uneven top line from withers to tail. As a breed, it has always been docile, gentle, and tractable.

Use

The Shetland Pony is mostly used as a pleasure animal for children, but is also seen in many show classes for riding and cart driving. As with all animals, it is important that it be properly trained to substantially increase its use as a pleasure mount for children.

Welsh Pony

The Welsh pony is native to the rough mountainous country of Wales. It is a very old breed, having been in existence for many centuries, probably since Saxon times in England.

It has been reported that in about 1825, a Thoroughbred stallion was turned loose among the bands of Welsh pony mares that ran wild in the more remote areas of the Welsh countryside. This Thoroughbred influence is traceable to the modern Welsh pony.

Characteristics

Height—10 to 14 hands. Colors—usually gray, roan, black, brown, or chestnut, though cream, dun, and white colors are found. In fact, any color other than the Pinto color is eligible for registry. White markings are not popular. The modern Welsh pony may be described as a miniature coach horse. It is bred to have a good head and neck, short coupling, and plenty of muscles and bone substance. It should also possess considerable speed and action at the trot and good endurance.

Use

The Welsh Pony's ruggedness and agility have made it useful as a child's riding mount, roadster, harness show pony, racing pony, trail pony, and parade pony. It is also used for stock cutting and hunting.

Pony of the Americas (POA)

The Pony of the Americas is, as the name indicates, a pony breed that originated in America. The registry was formed in 1954. The foundation stock came mostly from the breeding of the Appaloosa horse with the Welsh pony. A happy medium of Arabian and Quarter Horse type in miniature was sought and developed with the Appaloosa coloring.

Characteristics

Height—46 inches to 54 inches. If an individual does not fall into this size range at the age of six, it is disqualified for registry. Ponies that do not have the Appaloosa color are also disqualified.

Use

The Pony of the Americas is an all-around pleasure pony that was bred to meet the needs of the junior horseman who has outgrown Shetland ponies but who is not ready for horses.

2

Basic Considerations in the Care of the Horse

RESPONSIBILITIES OF THE HORSE OWNER

Owning a horse can be a wonderful experience and can open the door to untold hours of pleasure. It can offer children the opportunity to learn responsibilities, to enter the world of competition, to be introduced to the story of reproduction, and to enjoy an inner warm bond with his or her animal. Adults, too, can enjoy many of these experiences and find a world completely apart from their busy everyday worlds. It seems we must all find temporary escapes to be better able to appreciate the wonderful things of our lives—the beauty of trees and the evening sky.

However, with the ownership of a horse come certain responsibilities for the animal's care. These involve obtaining a basic knowledge of the horse's physical nature. It behooves all good horsemen not only to be equestrians but also to be good husbandrymen. A responsible horse owner is obligated to do the following:

1. Become familiar with the nature of horses and therefore understand basic safety rules for the horse and owner
2. Learn common terms to be able to "speak the language" of the horse world
3. Understand equine nutritional needs to provide a proper feeding program based on an animal's individual requirements
4. Provide good foot care and proper grooming

5. Know when a horse is healthy and when one is in bad condition (Figs. 2 and 3)
6. Obtain a knowledge of common diseases, their prevention, first-aid, and nursing
7. Understand proper wound care and first-aid
8. Be especially familiar with the parasite problem and routine dental care
9. Be familiar with the common types of lameness and unsoundness, their causes and prevention
10. Have a knowledge of the care of stallions, mares, and foals, and breeding physiology, if the owner is so involved
11. Learn when to call a veterinarian
12. Follow a check list (such as the one below) for good horse care:

Owners should provide:
1. Good and *safe* shelter, fences, and general surroundings
2. A good balanced feeding program
3. Plenty of clean water
4. Plenty of clean bedding if the horse is kept in a stall
5. Clean barn, corrals, or paddocks
6. Good foot care
7. Routine worming, vaccinations, and dental care
8. Frequent grooming

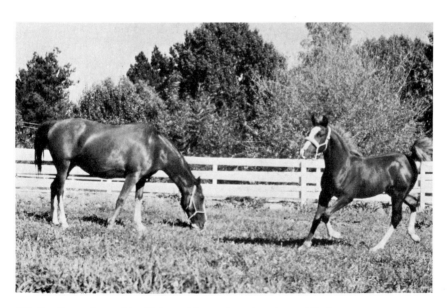

FIG. 2.   Horses in good health have shiny coats and are in good flesh.

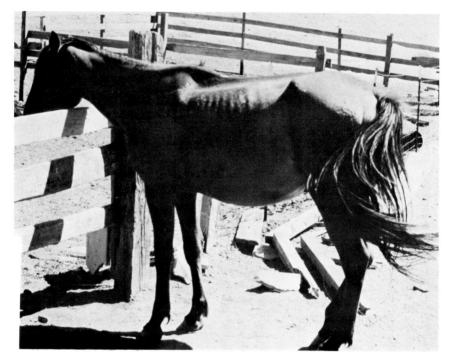

FIG. 3.   Horse in poor condition: ribs showing, with no flesh over withers or croup area.

    9. Consideration not to overwork or stress an uncon-
       ditioned animal
  10. True concern and compassion for the horse's well-
     being and a watchful eye to avoid situations most likely
     to result in problems.

SAFETY PRECAUTIONS

When handling a horse, you should be aware of the following
important safety precautions:
    1. Always warn a horse of your presence with a soft voice when
     approaching it from behind. Avoid making any sudden
     moves or noises that the horse does not expect.
    2. Work close to the horse. This will make it impossible for you
     to receive the full force of a kick. A spot close to the shoulder
     (preferably on the left) is the safest area to be standing when
     working around the animal. Avoid working directly in front
     or behind the horse.
    3. Never wrap a lead rope around your hand.
    4. Always give extra care not to startle a stallion.
    5. Be extra alert and cautious with a horse on windy days or

when using it after it has been restricted to a stall or small area for any prolonged period of time.
6. Avoid feeding a horse from your hand. This encourages butting and biting. Give treats in a bucket.

The following safety precautions should be taken to prevent a horse from injuring itself:
1. Provide safe stabling facilities. It is desirable to have a shelter area with at least three walls for horses to seek refuge from the elements. Have the area at least 12 × 12 foot for a single animal and twice that or larger if two or more animals are out together. This prevents an animal from getting cast (down too close to the walls to get up by himself) or too close quarters, which may cause fighting. Avoid sharp corners on feeders and water containers. Avoid low overhangs or protruding nails or bolts (Fig. 4). Keep junk and trash away from the horse. Have foolproof gate locks, preferably chained, to keep horses off roadways.
2. Keep grain securely locked away from horses. Horses overeat on grain if given the opportunity. Amounts of 25 pounds or more at one feeding can cause acute indigestion, colic, and

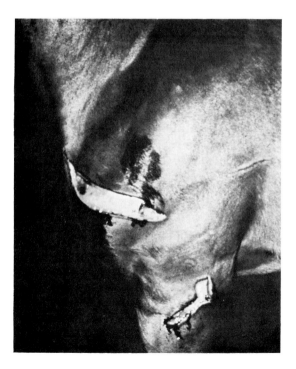

FIG. 4.   Injury caused by protruding nails in a barn.

even death. Foundering (laminitis), which can cause serious lameness, can be an aftermath.

3. Provide safe fencing. Eliminate barbed-wire fences if at all possible. They are frequently the most expensive type of fence when they cause serious injury to an animal (Figs. 5 and 6). A good wooden fence is often the most practical, although it requires frequent maintenance (Fig. 7). Chain-linked fence should either be buried six inches or left six inches above the ground to avoid horses getting a foot caught under them. Good pipe fences are perhaps best of all but require a significant investment. Steel posts for barbed-wire fences are dangerous, and if used, should be capped. It is desirable to fence off corners in corral areas when horses that fight are together.

4. Always tie a horse to a very secure object. Never tie a horse to a steel post that is just pounded into the ground or to a weak post. If frightened, it could pull up the post, run, and be impaled on the post.

5. Always tie a horse at shoulder height or higher, with no more than 18 to 24 inches of slack rope. If the rope is left long enough so that the animal's head can reach the ground,

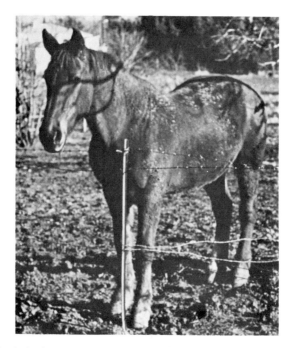

FIG. 5.   Barbed-wire fences cause many serious injuries to horses and often end up being the most expensive of all fences because of the losses they cause.

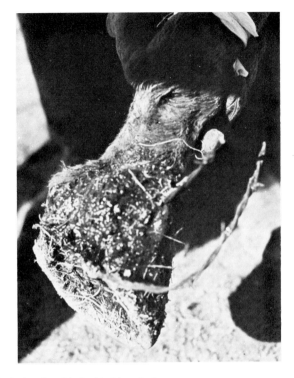

FIG. 6. Barbed-wire strand imbedded in a foot.

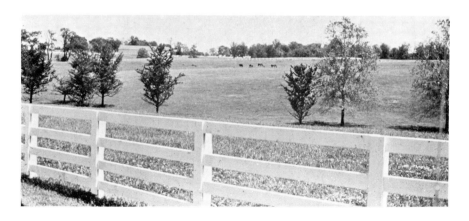

FIG. 7. A wood fence is often very satisfactory.

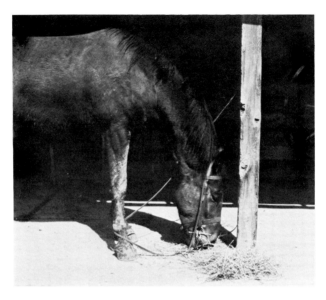

FIG. 8.   Never tie horse with long rope so that he can get his feet caught in the rope.

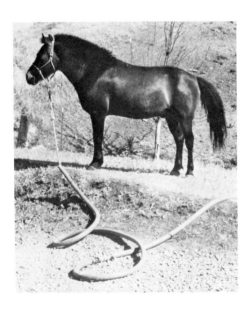

FIG. 9.   If a horse is to be tethered, it is wise to run the rope or chain through a garden hose to prevent severe rope burns.

he can easily get a foot tangled in it and get a severe rope burn or injury (Figs. 8 and 9). Tethering horses out to graze is a highly questionable procedure. Animals frequently get severe rope burns or break away to get out onto roads. Many horses become terrified when they feel a rope tangled about their feet, though some animals will stand for hours when hopelessly entangled in a rope or wire.

6. Never tie a horse "movie-cowboy style" by the reins. If it pulls back, the bit can cause injury to the mouth and the reins invariably break. Always carry a halter and lead rope with you to tie the animal.
7. Never tie a horse with a slip knot around its neck, no matter how gentle you may think it is. Choking can cause brain damage.
8. When removing a saddle with a double rigging, always remove the back cinch first. If this is not done, the horse may spook when the saddle is only half off, and the saddle will slip under it. This will cause it to panic, run, and often injure itself (besides damaging the saddle).

HANDLING TIPS

1. Groom a horse well before riding it, especially cleaning the back and feet thoroughly. This helps avoid irritation to the area under the saddle and helps prevent stone bruises to the feet.
2. Allow the horse to warm up before subjecting it to the exertion of a gallop or run.
3. When resting for lunch or any prolonged stop, loosen the cinch and recheck the horse's feet.
4. Bring the horse in cool by walking the last part of the ride. Always dry the animal and "cool him out" before putting it away after a hard ride or workout. Never feed grain to an animal that is hot or exhausted, or allow free drinking. Only allow a periodic small drink when cooling it down. Large quantities of water given to a hot animal can predispose it to founder; a grain feeding can cause serious indigestion, possible acute stomach swelling (gastric dilatation), and colic, which may be fatal. Good clean hay is always safe. Animals with long coats that are worked hard and work up a good sweat take a long time to cool out. It is a common practice to clip the body area (the legs and saddle area are left unclipped) to make it possible to cool these animals out faster. A clipped animal should have good shelter and should be blanketed at night to protect it from cold weather and chilling.

5. Never try to maintain your balance by pulling on the reins. It is best to grab for the saddle or mane. Such abuse to the horse's mouth can cause mouth injury and head tossing. Constant jerking on the horse's bit also tends to make it "hard-mouthed" and progressively more difficult to rein. It should be noted that wolf teeth (small premolar teeth located just in front of the first chewing teeth) are a common cause of head throwing. Not all horses have them and they should be checked for this by a veterinarian. If head tossing is a problem because of wolf teeth, the teeth often must be removed.
6. Regroom the animal after riding, taking special care to clean out the feet again.

PURCHASING A HORSE

When a family has decided to buy a horse, it is very important that the horse chosen be the "right one." Horses live a long time and frequently become very important members of a family. Purchasing an unsound or unsuitable horse can result in a great deal of unhappiness and often a significant financial loss. To avoid this, the following procedure and suggestions should be helpful.

When purchasing an animal, the buyer should not be too anxious. The following four steps should be the general plan: (1) survey the market; (2) screen the possibilities; (3) have the animal examined by a veterinarian; and (4) complete the purchase.

The Market

Horses can be purchased at breed sales or auctions or directly from breeders, dealers, or private parties.

Breed sales and dispersion sales are often excellent sources for quality animals. To guarantee soundness, most large sales have the animals examined by a veterinarian before the sale. On the other hand, open horse auctions and livestock auctions are risky places to purchase a horse. It is through these auctions that many individuals and dealers "dump" outlaws and unsound animals. Since the law says *caveat emptor* (buyer beware), one usually has no recourse if the horse purchased proves to be unsound.

Breeders are a good source for a specific type of horse. It is good to become familiar with the different breeds of horses and their various qualities. The public library will have books discussing this and will have addresses of the national headquarters of the breed associations. Through these associations, it is possible to obtain addresses of local breeders. Local feed stores and tack shops can also often supply this information.

Horse dealers can be a good source, but you should make many inquiries into the reputation of a given dealer before you deal with him.

Private parties are the most common sources for the purchase of pleasure horses. Many horses are advertised in local newspapers, in horse magazines, and on the bulletin boards of feed and saddle stores. Other leads may be obtained from local race tracks, trainers, riding stables, and breed and riding clubs.

Screening Possibilities

There are two major considerations in choosing a horse: price and suitability.

Price

Is the animal in the right price range? As with most purchases, you usually get what you pay for. The exact worth of a horse is often difficult to determine as it holds true that "a horse is worth what anyone is willing to pay for him." The following generalities may serve as broad guidelines: The average saddle horse is presently selling between $500 and $1000. There usually is a reason for a horse selling for $250 or less. Registered horses and those with exceptional beauty or training command prices from $1500 to $5000 or more. A common price range for good English-type horses is between $1500 and $10,000. Traditionally, Thoroughbreds and Arabians command high prices. Some individual horses have sold for over $1 million.

Suitability

Will this animal be the one you want to own? To determine this one should consider: looks and type; temperament; training; and age and soundness.

Looks. Does the animal appeal to you and is it the general type of animal in which you are interested? Though beauty is not a requisite for a good pleasure or performance horse, it can be an important feature of a show horse. If you are selecting a horse for breeding or for showing, it is advisable that you become familiar with breed and show standards regarding type and conformation.

In general, Quarter-type animals are most often used for Western riding. Thoroughbred-type horses are most often used for English riding, hunting, jumping, and dressage. Many can be used for any style riding. The size of the animal can also affect its suitability. It is always inadvisable to purchase too small an animal for a given rider. Small ponies, well-mannered, can be very suitable for young riders, but an adult's supervision is frequently required to remind the youngsters of their duties.

Temperament. This is perhaps the most important characteristic other than soundness to consider. No matter how beautiful or sound an animal is, if it is mean, has vicious habits, and is unpredictable, the horse is not worth having as a pleasure animal. This is especially true for the inexperienced or young rider. It can't be overemphasized how important it is to obtain a gentle, well-mannered animal for the novice rider. If a child develops fear early in his or her riding experience, he may lose complete interest and miss the many years of pleasure and sense of achievement known to an accomplished horseman. Unfortunately, temperament in a horse is next to impossible to change, though it is true that a highly nervous horse may perform well if it has developed confidence and security with its owner.

The following are some temperament tests that may give an insight to an individual animal:

On the ground
1. Is it hard to catch?
2. Does it appear nervous when approached?
3. Does it snort or prance about when you walk around it?
4. Does it resist having its feet picked up—front and back?
5. Does it lay its ears back or show any desire to bite or kick?

On horseback (it is best to have an experienced rider check the animal from the saddle)
1. Does the animal stand calmly or prance about?
2. Does it feel under control, both in a corral and in the open?
3. Does it shy easily? (Windy days make horses more nervous.)
4. How well does the animal respond to reining and leg aids?

Training. It is always unwise to purchase a green horse for an inexperienced rider and "let them learn together." This often results in the discouragement of the novice and may result in a disaster if the green horse is also highly spirited. The animal should have had basic training and should respond to the bit.

Training can be done by an inexperienced horseman with the aid of a good text. This in itself can be great fun, but it is important that the nature of the horse be understood. A horse needs to clearly understand what is expected of it before it is able to perform. A well-trained horse is the result of a great amount of patience and is a real pleasure to own.

Many horses require a professional trainer. Amazing results can be accomplished by a good trainer; but unfortunately, a bad temperament cannot be trained out of a given animal.

Age. The age of a horse need not be the major limiting factor at the time of purchase unless very special demands are to be made of the animal. The following remarks are generalities regarding the age of horses.

The average life expectancy for horses is between 25 and 30 years, although some have lived well past 35 years. One year of a horse's life is considered to be equal to about 3 years of a man's. For reasons not well understood, geriatric problems are not common. Many horses continue to act young right up to their last days, whereas others do show the effects of age. Chronic illnesses are relatively rare, except for arthritis.

HORSES AND THEIR USES AT DIFFERENT AGES. *1 week to 18 months.* At this time, early handling, halter breaking, and ground training are very beneficial. Studies in dogs and humans have indicated that basic personality and security are established in the first 6 weeks of life. If the foal develops an early sense of security with man, it may later prove to be more tractable and dependable. Since foals often pick up the mare's attitude toward man, it may be well to wean a foal early from a nervous, ill-tempered mare; however, evidence indicates that bad temperament is most likely inherited. Most colts are gelded between 8 and 18 months, but it may be done at a later age if the colt is not too fractious.

18 months to 3 years. Early basic training is given at this time. If the animal is well developed, much of this training can be done from the saddle. Racing of 2-year-olds is the common practice, but due to their immaturity, 60% of the 2-year-olds break down at the track. It is very important not to rush these young animals by hard work. It is usually best to wait until the animals are 3-year-olds before they are used for breeding. A good feeding and worming program pays particularly high dividends in this age group.

3 to 5 years. Horses usually reach their mature size at 4 years of age, but some of their bones are not fused (closed epiphyseal plates) until they are nearly 7. This is why it is not advisable to jump these young animals, although they may be used fairly freely as pleasure horses. Few race horses compete past this age period.

6 to 12 years. Horses at this age are in their prime and can, with proper training and conditioning, be used for any standard horse activity.

12 to 20 years. Since aging problems are relatively uncommon, horses in this age group are rarely limited in their normal activities. It should be pointed out and emphasized that horses are not "over the hump" and ready for the glue factory at 15. It is the rule rather than the exception that these animals have 10 years or more of dependable serviceability to give.

20 to 25 years. These horses are often very suitable as mounts for children and are not necessarily limited in their usability because of age. They frequently have mellowed to the ways of man and are very dependable. Unfortunately, this is not always the case. A good dependable horse can do wonders for the development of a young rider's confidence. It is not uncommon for horses of this age to still be winning blue ribbons.

25 to 30 years. Though it is true that many horses will act like 10-year-olds until their last days, it should be realized that dental, digestive, tumor, and arthritic problems are not uncommon in this age group. Although it may continue to retain its youthful attitudes, it is only wise to show respect for the aged horse. These animals usually do need additional care and should not just be "turned out to pasture" to die. Too often, this means 40 acres of dirt for them to make out the best they can. This is cruel and inhumane, and it should be seen that their needs (more easily digested feed, protection, dental care, etc.) are met. Though these horses do often serve well as children's horses, the emotional experience of losing this pet in the not too distant future must be weighed.

Veterinary Examination

After an animal that seems suitable in all respects has been found, it is advisable to have a veterinarian examine it for soundness. The horse is examined for general health and soundness of heart, lungs, eyes, and legs. Blemishes are noted, if any are present, and the animal is examined for any evidence of lameness. The horse's age is also determined. From his findings and experience, and his noting of temperament, the veterinarian will give a professional opinion as to the condition, soundness, and suitability of the animal for the intended rider and the horse's intended use. The use of radiographs for a prepurchase examination is of value if the animal is meant to be used extensively as a jumper. It may be possible to detect early signs of arthritis that are not otherwise apparent. The clinical findings at the time of the examination give the best indication of the animal's present state of health and soundness.

Prepurchase examinations by veterinarians are a common procedure and are accepted by all horse people. It does not denote a sign of distrust between the buyer and the seller. Most sellers encourage this examination because it settles the question of the animal's soundness at the time of sale. It is wise to be cautious if there is pressure for a quick sale without time for an examination. If the seller is of good will and wants to rush the sale, he will accept a qualified endorsed check, "For _____ animal upon being found sound by a veterinarian's examination."

As a rule, it is best to have the examination made on the owner's property before the animal is moved. This will eliminate any question about soundness before the animal was moved. It should be noted that a veterinary examination is a service performed for the potential buyer, so he should be the one to contact the veterinarian directly as well as the one to pay for the service. This service may be instrumental in avoiding much unhappiness, disappointment, and financial loss. Always be well advised and not too anxious before making a purchase. Horses live a long time, so make a good, careful choice.

Complete the Purchase

When, finally, it has been decided that a given animal is "the right one," the purchase should be concluded in a businesslike manner, leaving no misunderstandings. For the agreed-upon price, if paid in full, the buyer should receive a bill of sale stating the name of the buyer, a description of the horse, and the terms of the purchase (price); this should be signed by the seller. If the animal is to be purchased by scheduled payments, the terms of the agreement should be stated and signed by both parties, a copy of which is kept by both buyer and seller. If the horse is registered, and the price is based on this registration, these papers should be signed over at the time the animal is paid for in full. If the papers are not immediately available, it is advisable to withhold part of the purchase price until they are available. The validity and value of the registration papers should be determined before a higher price is paid for the animal.

EQUINE HEALTH INSURANCE

Most horse insurance policies are written to protect the owner's investment in case of death from any cause not excluded in the policy. They also allow for voluntary destruction for humane considerations. These policies are, in effect, *life insurance* on valuable animals. It is unfortunate that most policies are so written that, in case of a serious injury, the animal must be euthanized in order for the owner to collect on the policy. They do not provide compensation for the reduced value of that animal in the event that the animal received treatment and recovered but did not regain its prior serviceability.

There is *surgical insurance* available to cover horses that may require major emergency surgery (e.g., for colic). Since successful abdominal surgery, although expensive, is common today, such a policy should be given serious consideration for valuable purebreds and performance animals, as well as for beloved companion mounts. Though equine health insurance policies to cover the treatment of illnesses were at one time available, the author does not know whether they still are, nor how practical such policies were.

The best equine health insurance a horse owner can get, in the opinion of the author, is a good personal relationship with the local equine veterinarian. Owners should call the veterinarian for such routine services as vaccinations, dental care, and parasite control. This allows the veterinarian to become familiar with the owner and the horse(s) and allows the owner to know how best to locate the veterinarian in an emergency. This knowledge helps the veterinarian to provide more efficient emergency service, which could make the difference between an uneventful recovery and a tragedy. Making this effort to know one's local veterinarian is the owner's *least expensive horse health insurance.*

AGING A HORSE

Horses' teeth (Fig. 10) continue to grow throughout their lives and wear in characteristic ways. Because of this, their front teeth (incisors) are readily available calendars that attest to the animal's age. With experience and practice, it is possible to determine a horse's age up to 30 years, fairly accurately, within a year or two. Fortunately, these changes that occur do so in a manner that is easy to memorize and that can be learned without much difficulty.

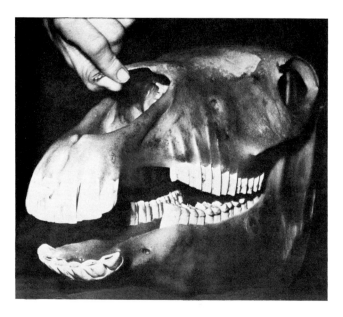

FIG. 10.　Sharp points cut into cheeks and tongue.

ERUPTION OF PERMANENT INCISORS

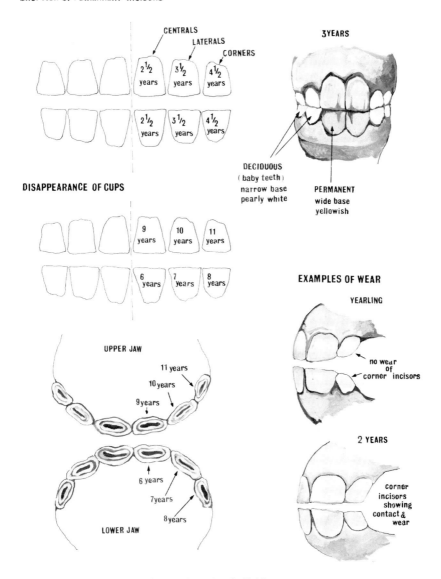

CHART I.   Aging horses. (Drawings by Jeannine Quilici.)

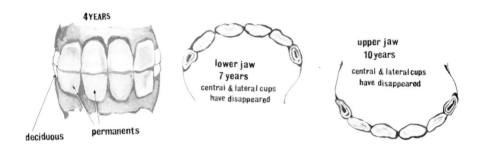

4 YEARS

deciduous   permanents

**lower jaw
7 years**
central & lateral cups
have disappeared

**upper jaw
10 years**
central & lateral cups
have disappeared

GALVAYNE'S GROOVE

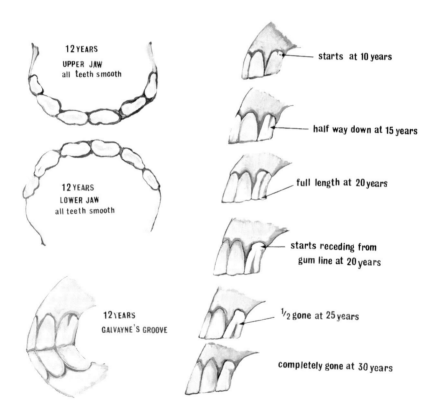

**12 YEARS
UPPER JAW**
all teeth smooth

**12 YEARS
LOWER JAW**
all teeth smooth

**12 YEARS
GALVAYNE'S GROOVE**

starts at 10 years

half way down at 15 years

full length at 20 years

starts receding from
gum line at 20 years

½ gone at 25 years

completely gone at 30 years

SHAPE CHANGE OF CHEWING SURFACES OF LOWER INCISORS

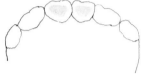

central incisors triangular at 16 years

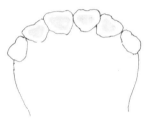

lateral incisors triangular at 17 years

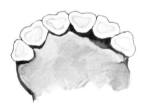

corner incisors triangular at 18 years

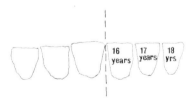

The aging technique is based on three groups of dental changes: (1) eruption of permanent incisors, (2) disappearance of cups, and (3) the development and disappearance of Galvayne's groove.

Eruption of Permanent Incisors

There are three pairs of lower and upper incisors. They are referred to as centrals, laterals, and corners, from the midline outward. Temporary incisors, which have a narrow base at the gum line and are pearly white (Fig. 11), are replaced by permanent incisors (Fig. 12), which are larger and darker and have a wide base, in the following order:

2½ years . . . . centrals (both upper and lower)
3½ years . . . . laterals (both upper and lower)
4½ years . . . . corners (both upper and lower)
5 years . . . . bridle teeth (canines) in males only

Disappearance of Cups

The chewing surfaces of the incisors show cups (dark holes) until they are worn smooth (Fig. 13). Very conveniently, the cups disappear in an orderly manner, as follows:

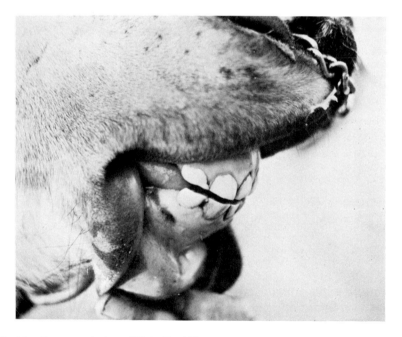

FIG. 11. Temporary incisors ("Baby Teeth") are pearly white and smaller than permanent incisors.

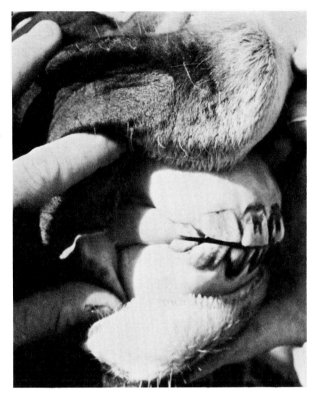

FIG. 12. This horse is four years old. The permanent corner incisors have not come in yet, which happens at four and one-half years.

6 years .... central lowers
7 years .... lateral lowers
8 years .... corner lowers
9 years .... central uppers
10 years .... lateral uppers
11 years .... corner uppers

Thus an 11-year-old horse is referred to as "smooth mouthed."

Galvayne's Groove

This is a groove that occurs in the upper corner incisors only. It first appears at the gum line at 10 years of age. It then seems to work its way downward as the tooth wears. At 20 years, Galvayne's groove extends the full length of the tooth. When it is halfway down, the animal is 15 and variation therein can be judged. At age 20 the groove begins to disappear at the gum line

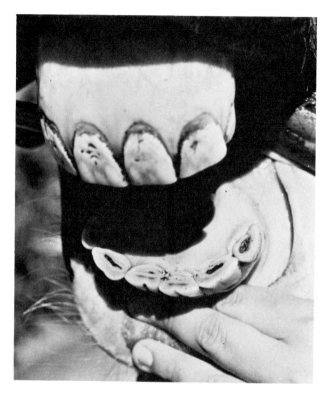

FIG. 13. "Cups" are present in the lower lateral and corner incisors, but are gone from the centrals, thus the horse is six years old.

and is completely gone at age 30. When only the lower half of the tooth manifests the groove, the animal is 25 (Fig. 14). Likewise, variations in the length of the groove that remains give an indication of the horse's age. It should be noted that there may occasionally be a slight difference in the length of the groove from the right to the left side of the mouth. An in-between-age estimation will be close.

A 2-year-old can be distinguished from a yearling by the wear shown on the corner temporary incisors. These uppers and lowers have not met in yearlings.

The chewing surfaces of the lower incisors become triangular in shape at the following ages (Fig. 15):

16 years . . . . centrals triangular
17 years . . . . laterals triangular
18 years . . . . corners triangular

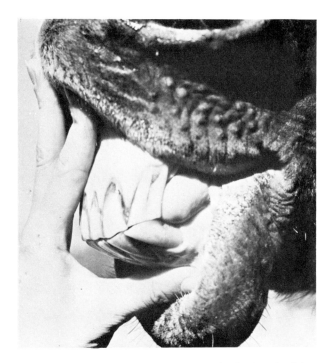

FIG. 14. Galvayne's groove is almost completely down the full length of the upper corner incisor, thus the horse is approximately nineteen years old.

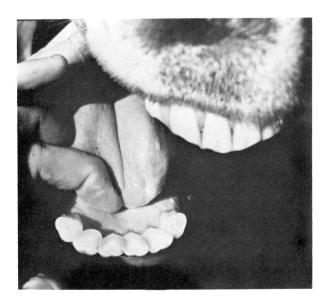

FIG. 15. All bottom incisors are triangular in shape, thus the horse is eighteen or over.

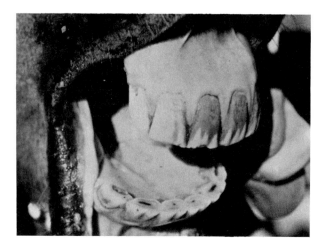

FIG. 16. An unusual horse that has the cups of a seven-year-old but the Galvayne's groove of a twelve-year-old. The groove is the more accurate.

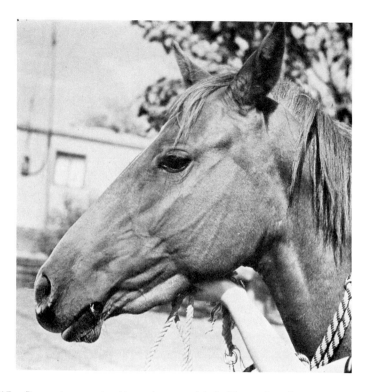

FIG. 17. Bony enlargements of lower jaw associated with eruption of permanent teeth.

Over 90% of horses consistently show these overall dental changes. The most common variation is the retention of cups, which seems to be dependent upon the ration received. An individual animal may show the cups of an 8-year-old, but have a Galvayne's groove that indicates an age of 14. Changes in the groove seem most consistent, but an educated guess taking into account overall dental changes (Figs. 16 and 17) may be necessary.

CHAPTER

3

Unsoundness

A horse is considered *sound* when the animal has no condition that interferes with its intended use. An abnormal condition that does interfere with the animal's serviceability is called an *unsoundness*. It should be noted that the state of soundness is not constant. Many injuries can cause temporary unsoundness and may be of only minor concern. On the other hand, many problems can render the animal permanently unsound for certain types of use. A veterinarian can best evaluate the seriousness and prognosis of different types of unsoundness. As a general rule, it is always unwise to purchase an unsound horse, even though the unsoundness may appear to be temporary, such as an illness. Too commonly, conditions that seem temporary can be serious or mask a more serious problem.

Although many injuries can result in *blemishes* that do not interfere with the usefulness of a horse, certain *vices*, or bad habits, can definitely make the animal undesirable, dangerous, and no pleasure to own. Such conditions are as important as the physical state of the horse, if the horse is to be of any pleasure to the owner.

LAMENESS

Lameness is the major cause for unsoundness in the horse. The old adage, "no foot, no horse," is just as true today as ever. A lameness is a departure from the normal stance or gait, caused by disease or injury. It is a symptom of a problem. Although pain is the cause for 90% of the signs of lameness, some anatomical changes that do not cause pain can result in "mechanical lameness." Such conditions are not physically distressing to the animal. Painful lamenesses are more pronounced after exercise, either immediately or the next day. Because most lamenesses are the result of pain, it is difficult to justify using a lame horse for work or pleasure. Too often, this is done because the horse makes no noise to indicate the pain he is suffering.

The *signs of lameness* vary with the severity and nature of the problem. *Limping* is the result of lameness and such a statement as "He just limps a little; he isn't really lame" is contradictory. The trot is the best gait at which to detect a lameness. This causes extra concussion on the legs. Circling a horse in a relatively small circle (30 to 40 feet in diameter) at the trot is very helpful to demonstrate a lameness and to indicate which foot or leg is affected. The affected leg will usually take a shorter stride and be accompanied by a quickened effort to get weight off the leg. *Head bobbing* is a sign of front-leg lameness (the head comes up as the lame foot hits the ground), and a *dropping of the hip* is a sign of a hind-leg lameness.

Pointing is the action of a horse at rest who extends one front foot out in front of the other, which indicates that that foot is painful to him (Fig. 18). Although it is normal for a horse to alternate resting its hind feet, such action with the front feet is not normal and indicates a problem.

Stiffness in the front feet is evident when the horse shows re-

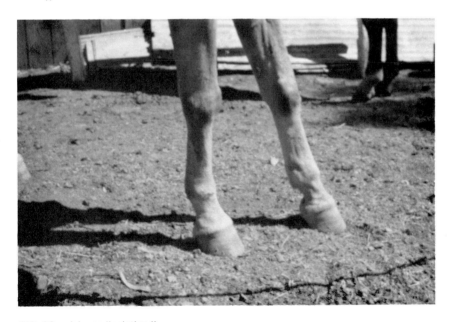

FIG. 18.   A horse "pointing."

luctance to move out freely when asked to trot. If both front feet are very painful, the horse will frequently stand with its hind feet well underneath him and its front feet out in front as much as possible. This is very characteristic of a horse with laminitis. Stiffness in older horses is often due to arthritis. There are only two common conditions that cause lameness in both front feet at the same time: navicular disease and laminitis. Pointing is most often a sign seen with navicular disease, and the painful "walking on eggs" gait is usually characteristic of laminitis. A very strong digital pulse in both front feet is found in laminitis, but not in navicular disease. The *digital pulse* is felt just below the fetlock, deep in the grooves between the pastern bones and the flexor tendons running behind the pastern. The pulse is felt by pressing firmly into both the inside and outside grooves using the thumb and the middle finger of one hand, both at the same time. Normally, a digital pulse is almost imperceptible. Any acute inflammation in the hoof causes a very strong pounding digital pulse. When a strong pulse is found in both front feet, the horse most likely has laminitis. If only one foot has a strong pulse, accompanied by a lameness in that leg, the cause of the lameness can be attributed to an inflammation in that hoof. Nail punctures, local infection, deep thrush, or stone bruises are common causes for a foot with a strong unilateral (only one front foot) digital pulse. It should be noted that 80% of all lamenesses originate in the hoof, even though it may appear to the inexperienced horseman to be from the shoulder. Shoulder lameness is very rare.

Causes of Lameness

The causes of lameness are many. Though many lamenesses result from accidental injuries, there are many factors that predispose a horse to lameness. These factors include the following: immaturity for hard work (e.g., racing 2-year-olds), faulty conformation, general poor condition or conditioning, nutritional deficiencies or imbalances, fatigue, bad shoeing, lack of attention to the feet, illness, and local leg infections.

It is of interest to note that, of 2-year-olds that race, more than 60% break down. These young animals don't even have a 50/50 chance of surviving the rigors of the stresses and strains of racing—all this for man's glory and his pocketbook. There is much evidence that if racing could be delayed until the horses were 30 months old, most such losses could be eliminated.

In the pleasure horse, the most common immediate causes of lameness include stone bruises, hoof puncture wounds, other hoof and leg wounds, sprains, navicular disease, tendonitis (from over-stretching the tendons), laminitis, tender feet from trimming too closely, and thrush. Less frequent but not too uncommon causes include ring bone, bowed tendons, stifle, and fractures.

Race horses are more commonly afflicted with such conditions as: bruised soles, bowed tendons, bucked shins, osselets, popped knees (carpitis with or without bone chips), fractured sesamoid bone in the fetlocks, and other fractures.

Stone Bruise

A stone bruise to the sole of the hoof is one of the most common causes of lameness in the pleasure horse. Running the horse along sides of black top or gravel roads or over rough, rocky terrain predisposes the animal to this problem. The lameness will most often have a sudden onset. The degree of lameness will vary with the severity of the bruise. A strong digital pulse along with a noticeable tender area detected with a hoof tester are characteristic findings. There normally is no swelling of the leg. First-aid treatment of soaking the foot in a bucket of ice water or standing the horse in mud is indicated. The possibility of a hoof puncture or "graveled" should be eliminated before using the mud treatment. The ice bucket method is safe in all cases. The use of aspirin in the grain is also useful to reduce local inflammation (50 g twice daily in grain). It is advisable, especially if the lameness is severe, to have a veterinarian make the proper diagnosis so a specific and effective treatment program can be started. The use of anti-inflammatory drugs is very useful for the treatment of stone bruises. Their use can greatly shorten the recovery period and result in less damage to the foot.

Hoof Puncture Wounds

The seriousness of this problem can vary greatly, depending on the specific structures affected in the hoof, the degree of damage, and the presence of infection.

Signs. Acute lameness most often accompanies a hoof puncture if the puncture is into the sensitive part of the hoof. A marked posterior digital pulse will be present. Often the nail or other object is present when the foot is examined. If not, one can usually find the entrance of the puncture into the sole or crevice of the frog by cutting down to a clean sole structure with a hoof knife, looking for a black hole to follow down. A hoof tester is often helpful to pinpoint a tender location. If the puncture went into the soft frog, most often the hole will not be found because holes in the frog have a tendency to seal over rapidly, like a nail puncture in a rubber tire. If the injury is old and an infection has entered the foot, a black pus-like discharge will be reached if the track is followed down to the infection inside and under the sole, and opened to establish drainage.

Procedure. A horse with a puncture wound should receive tetanus protection. Antibiotics should be given to prevent or treat infection. If a nail or object is removed, the wound hole can be treated with an antibiotic ointment, Kopertox, or tincture of iodine. This is one of the few kinds of wounds in which one can use a drying astringent-type wound dressing in a deep wound. The use of aspirin is recommended to minimize inflammation and pain. If the condition worsens or shows no improvement in 24 to 48 hours after its initial treatment, then hot epsom-salts soaking may be necessary to help establish drainage from the site of the infection. The author prefers not to have to open the sole unless necessary because it takes some time for the sole to grow out. Stubborn infections should be treated diligently with the heavy doses of antibiotics.

Gravel

A horse is said to have "graveled" when an infection has worked up into the foot from the sole at the junction of the sole and the hoof wall. Severe lameness results. This is one of the common causes of lameness. Treatment is directed toward trying to establish drainage, use of antibiotics, and tetanus protection. An abscess pocket under the sole can be mechanically drained by cutting down into the area with a hoof knife. Characteristically, the drainage from such an abscess is blackish and the opening of the abscess gives immediate release of pressure and relief to this very painful condition. Occasionally, the infection may work upward and drain out up above along the coronet. The condition can be initially diagnosed by noting acute lameness to the affected foot, a strong digital pulse, marked pain to a hoof tester (pincher) over the affected area, and a small, black crack that is noted to continue deep into the foot as the area is pared away with a hoof knife. Most often, complete recovery occurs after the condition has had the proper treatment that is necessary to limit this infection.

Navicular Disease

Navicular disease is a common cause of equine lameness. This condition affects both front feet at the same time. It begins as a soft tissue bursitis in the navicular bursa deep in the foot under the frog. In time, it develops into a progressive degenerative arthritis. Horses as young as 4 years old can be affected, but the disease is most common in horses over 7 years of age.

The exact cause is not known, but possible factors are continuous concussion, especially on hard surfaces; very straight pastern conformation, which may be hereditary; and poor shoeing or trimming, which does not allow for normal frog pressure and thus normal circulation. Normal circulation is necessary to maintain good hoof elasticity, which is necessary for good shock absorption function of the hoof. Without this, the frog and the deep structures under it can receive continuous jolting when the animal is worked. This can be especially important to horses used for jumping.

Symptoms. Most horses with navicular disease display a characteristic pattern of behavior before persistent lameness occurs. The onset is insidious, that is, the disease progresses slowly and is not characterized by a sudden lameness. Owners first may notice that the horse stumbles for no apparent reason, or may seem stiff going downhill. This may go away for a time, but it often reappears. The horse may then go lame for short periods and then recover. Weeks may go by before any further signs are noticed. This initial lameness may appear as a stiffness in the front legs or as an actual lameness in one foot. The lameness may seem to occasionally shift from one leg to the other. With time, perhaps months, the lameness progresses until the animal appears lame all the time. In the early stages, exercise causes the animal to "warm out" of the lameness, but the animal is usually extra stiff the following day.

Diagnosis. Because the disease is initially a soft tissue disease problem, radiographs are of no help in early cases, but are useful in chronic cases in confirming the diagnosis.

The most effective way of diagnosing navicular disease is to use a local anesthetic injected over the nerves going to the navicular area. This is referred to by veterinarians as a diagnostic bilateral posterior digital nerve block. This just blocks out the feelings in the back one-third of the foot, stopping any pain coming from the navicular area. The nerve blocking is done to both front feet. If lameness seems very evident in just one foot, nerve blocking that foot alone will only shift the lameness to the other foot. This is because in some cases one foot will hurt more than the other, but once the pain is gone from that foot, the animal will show lameness in the other foot. The nerve blocking is used because it is impossible to know exactly where the horse hurts. If the horse has navicular disease, it stops limping or showing stiffness and moves out freely within 5 to 10 minutes. This freedom from pain only lasts about 4 hours, after which time the lameness recurs because the nerve block has worn off.

Treatment. No way has been found to cure navicular disease. Drug therapy and corrective shoes only offer temporary relief. To

date, the most effective treatment for navicular disease is surgery
(Fig. 19). Fortunately, the anatomy of the nerve supply to the
navicular area makes it possible to short-circuit these nerve pathways of pain to the brain without disturbing the mechanical function or health of other important structures in the foot. The surgical technique involves removing a segment of the nerves (there
are two major nerve trunks to each foot) that supply the diseased
area. This is done just below the fetlock. Small nerve branches
are also removed if they are present (they are present in about
70% of the horses). The surgery is effective in about 80% of the
cases. The reason why this procedure is not 100% effective is not
clear.

When the surgery is completely effective, the animal is usually
free from the lameness of navicular disease for life. Such "nerved"
horses need not be restricted in any way. They can be used safely

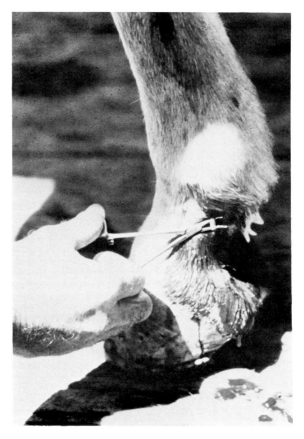

FIG. 19.   Surgery being performed for navicular disease. The surgery is about 80% successful
and is the best method to get lasting results for this disease.

for racing, jumping, working, or pleasure riding. Since surgery is the only therapy for a condition that causes permanent, painful lameness if it remains untreated, the procedure is common practice and in itself causes no harm, but corrective shoes should be tried first.

Bowed Tendons (Tendonitis)

Overstretching of the flexor tendons of one or both front legs can cause a breakdown or rupture of the tendon fibers and local blood vessels. This causes acute inflammation of the tissues. The degree of inflammation is directly related to the amount of damage that has occurred. Severe tissue damage results in a great amount of local tissue reaction, scar tissue formation, and adhesions.

Common predisposing factors are overexertion without proper conditioning, strenuous work at too early an age, fatigue, continued work after first signs of tendon soreness have appeared, working on too hard a surface or strenuous work in deep mud, toes that are allowed to grow too long, and poor conformation (pasterns being too long).

Signs. The horse suddenly becomes acutely lame and attempts to stand with its heel off the ground. The tendons that are behind the cannon bone are sensitive to local pressure, feel warm, and are swollen. Long-standing cases show scar tissue, which causes the tendons to be thicker and appear "bowed" out from the leg. In old cases where the condition has "set" or cooled out completely and healed fairly well, no lameness may be observed. The damaged tendon, which can never be as strong as it was before the disease, rarely holds up under very strenuous work. Many of these horses can withstand hunting and jumping activities, taking 3½-foot fences without causing renewed damage to the legs, but this is not true in every case, and extra care is always in order.

Treatment. Tendonitis is most effectively treated in the early stages, before much scar tissue (fibrotic granulation tissue) has had a chance to develop. It is this tissue that causes further weakening and restriction of the tendons from adhesions. Ice packs should be applied as early as possible for 20 to 30 minutes as a first-aid measure. The leg should then be padded well and wrapped securely with a supportive bandage until a veterinarian can be called to treat the case.

The veterinarian applies either a plaster cast or a gelatin supportive bandage (flexible cast) to immobilize the damaged area as quickly as possible. If the injury is extensive, he may inject cortisone drugs directly into the injured area as well as into the blood to work systemically. It is very important to minimize the inflammation in the tendon to reduce the possible buildup of the scar tissue that is so damaging. The use of DMSO can be helpful.

After the plaster or flexible cast is removed, the animal should be given at least another 4 to 6 weeks of rest with only light exercise. Supportive bandages may be needed during this recovery period.

Older cases that have cooled out and are still showing lameness may be candidates for the tendon-splitting surgical procedure, which often allows freer movement and promotes normal action of the tendons. Such injured tendons never regain their original elasticity and tensile strength. Firing and blistering are methods of treatment that seldom if ever benefit a case and may cause more damage to the tissues. Firing neither welds the tissues back together nor makes them stronger than normal tendons.

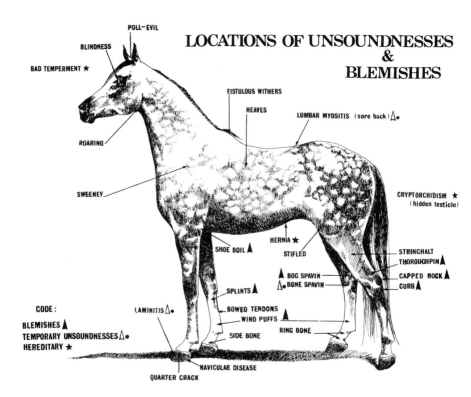

FIG. 20. Locations of unsoundnesses and blemishes. (Drawing by Jeannine Quilici.)

CHART I. Unsoundnesses and Blemishes

		UNSOUNDNESS	BLEMISH	COMMON	UNCOMMON	SERIOUS	SELDOM CAUSES LAMENESS	CAUSES LAMENESS	HEREDITARY PREDISPOSITION	NUTRITION POSSIBLE FACTOR
(A) HEAD	POLL EVIL	×				×	×			
	BLINDNESS	×			×	×				
(B) WITHERS & SHOULDER	FISTULOUS WITHERS	×				×	×			
	SWEENEY		×			×	×	±		
(C) FRONT LEGS	SHOE BOIL		×			×	×			
	SPLINTS		×	×			×			×
	BOWED TENDONS	×			×		×	×		
	WIND PUFFS		×	×			×			
	RINGBONE	×			×		×	×	- × -	×
	SIDEBONE		×	×			×		- × -	×
(D) FEET	LAMINITIS	×			×		×	×		×
	NAVICULAR DISEASE	×			×		×	×	- × -	×
(E) REAR LEGS	BOG SPAVIN	±	×	×			×			
	BONE SPAVIN	×				×		×	×	×
	THOROUGHPIN		×			×	×			
	CURB		×			×	×		- × -	
	STRINGHALT	×				×	×	×		
(F) GENERAL	HEAVES	×				×	×			×
	ROARING	×				×	×			
	HERNIA ·	±				×	±		×	
	SORE BACK	±		×			±	×		×
	BAD TEMPERAMENT	×			×		×		×	×

- × - because of conformation cryptorchidism and malocclusions are hereditary.

53

SPECIFIC LOCATIONS OF UNSOUNDNESSES (Fig. 20)

Head

Defective eyes, such as blindness, extensive cornea scars, or tumors may affect a horse's dependability and usability.

Poll evil is a serious infection of the bursa of the poll and is almost impossible to cure. Fortunately, it is a rare condition.

Withers and Shoulders

Fistulous withers (Fig. 21) is a serious infection of the bursa over the withers. Like poll evil, it is almost incurable. Radical surgery is sometimes effective.

Sweeney (Fig. 22) is a depression above the shoulder due to atrophied muscles caused by a nerve injury at the point of the shoulder. It is only an unsoundness if it causes lameness.

Front Legs and Feet

Bowed tendons are enlarged flexor tendons behind the cannon bones that have resulted from overstretching or tearing of the tendons or tendon sheaths. The condition may occur in one or both front legs, and occasionally occurs in the hind legs. It is the most common cause of permanent retirement of race horses. Once these tendons have "set," often taking over a year, and no lameness is present, many of these animals may stay sound for many uses. Very hard work, such as open jumping or steeplechasing, will likely cause reinjury and lameness.

Laminitis (founder) is an inflammation of the sensitive laminae just under the wall of the hooves. Because the hoof wall does not expand, the inflamed tissue is under increased pressure. This

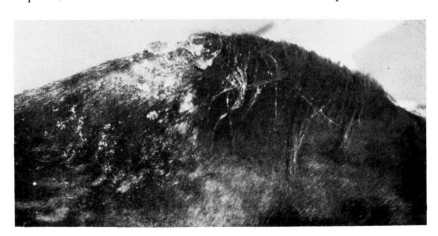

FIG. 21. Fistulous withers.

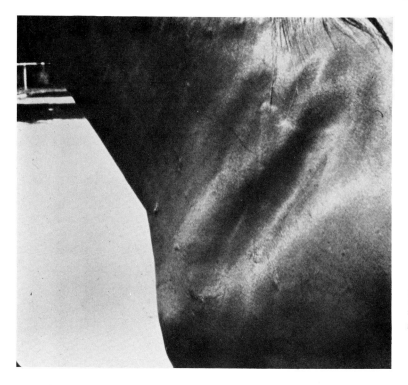

FIG. 22. Sweeney. (Courtesy of Dr. Pierre Lieux, Riverside, CA.)

results in a very painful condition. Laminitis is common and animals that have suffered with the problem are more susceptible to recurrence. However, the degree of susceptibility depends on the initial cause.

Navicular disease is an inflammation of the small navicular bone and bursa of the front feet. It is a common cause of lameness and develops into a progressive arthritis (see previous discussion).

Ringbone is a calcium deposit that frequently encircles the pastern bones of the front feet. It may occur in the hind legs, where it is usually the result of direct injury. Short, straight pasterns and work on hard surfaces predispose the horse to this common (and very serious) disease. The use of cortisone drugs injected directly into the enlargement is sometimes helpful. Ringbone is a common cause of permanent lameness (Figs. 23 and 24).

Sidebones are calcified lateral cartilages of the front feet (Fig. 25). These structures are normally involved in the shock absorption function of the hoof. They are caused by work on hard surfaces. Usually, they do not cause lameness. Special shoeing is often used to treat sidebones, and side grooving of the hoof is also occasionally effective.

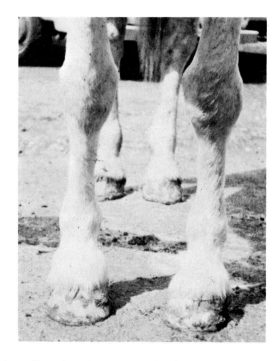

FIG. 23.   Ringbone. The enlarged pastern area (calcium deposits) is characteristic.

Hind Legs and Feet

Stifled is a condition in which the patella (knee cap) catches under one of its ligaments. This causes the animal to drag its hind foot on the toe because it is unable to advance it normally. If the animal is forced to back up, the knee cap will pop back into place. The horse can then move forward normally. Forced stall rest for 7 to 10 days with the use of aspirin twice daily in the grain is helpful. If the condition constantly recurs, surgery can correct the problem. It is common in ponies and is predisposed by straight stifle joints. The injection of a sclorosing agent over the affected ligament is sometimes helpful.

Bone spavin is a bony enlargement (calcium deposit) low on the inside of the hock (Fig. 26). It usually does not cause permanent lameness, but it may.

Stringhalt is a peculiar jerking up of the hind legs at the walk or trot. The cause is unknown, but nerve degeneration may be a cause. Surgery frequently helps.

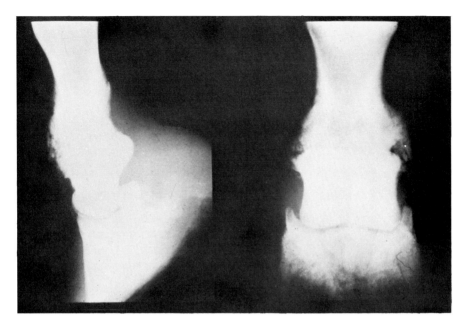

FIG. 24. X-ray of case of ringbone. Tendons rubbing against the calcium deposits cause pain and lameness.

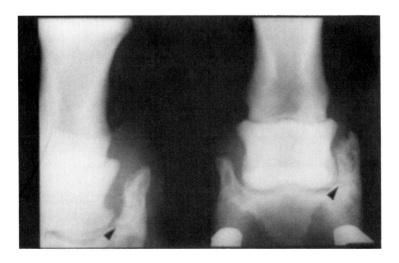

FIG. 25. X-ray of sidebones.

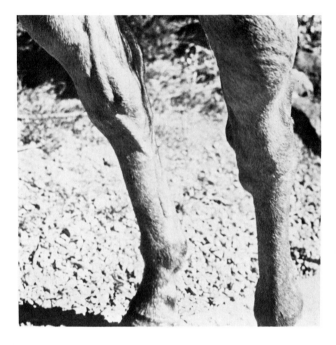

FIG. 26.   Bone spavin is a calcium enlargement low on the inside of the hock.

GENERAL UNSOUNDNESSES

Heaves (broken wind or emphysema) is a permanent condition resulting from the breakdown of lung tissue. Wheezing and difficult breathing are the usual symptoms. It most often results from an untreated, prolonged chronic cough. Certain allergies may bring on marked symptoms. The reduced lung capacity makes it necessary for the animal to use more of his abdominal muscles for breathing. The constant use of the abdominal muscles results in a visible muscular ridge seen in the flank area which is called the "heaveline." Affected animals have very little stamina and are not useful for riding.

It should be noted that horses are sometimes affected by acute attacks of "hay fever" (allergic respiratory congestion), which can develop into serious asthma (Fig. 27). Such horses might at first be thought to be suffering from the more permanent condition of emphysema. These asthma attacks result in extensive lung congestion, which causes very labored breathing, wheezing, and often anoxia (deficiency of oxygen). Such cases need immediate medical attention and are usually successfully treated with corticosteroids or antihistamines. Untreated horses may die. Forced exercise during an acute attack can very easily cause death. Those

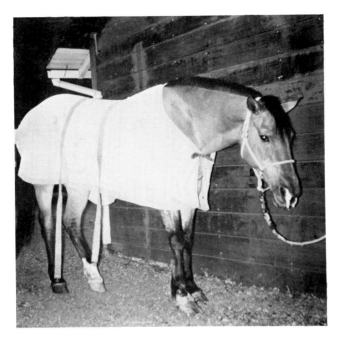

FIG. 27.   Horse having an acute asthma attack. Prompt treatment is indicated.

that recover do so fully and may not be affected again for months or years.

Roaring is a condition that causes an abnormal sound heard on expiration. It is the result of a nerve paralysis to the laryngeal saccule in the larynx. With no normal nerve supply, the saccule loses its normal tension, and flutters as the air passes out of the lungs causing the characteristic "roaring" sound. This reduces efficient breathing and stamina. Surgery can correct this.

Hernia, also referred to as a rupture, is a protrusion of tissue through an abdominal opening. Two common hernias occur in the horse, umbilical and scrotal. Both are hereditary. *Scrotal hernias* occur inside the scrotum and are occasionally seen at birth in the stud colt, but are rarely large enough to require surgical repair. At times, physical replacement of the tissue back up through the inguinal ring is necessary. This procedure may have to be repeated several times during the first few days of life, after which the condition often is self-corrected.

Umbilical hernias at the naval area are much more common and occur in either sex (Fig. 28). Most of these correct themselves by the time the animal is a yearling. Rarely is surgery done before this age unless the hernia is large and there is a significant chance that the tissue (which can include a loop of intestine in a large

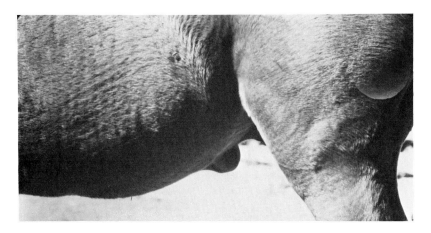

FIG. 28. Umbilical hernia.

hernia) may become strangulated when this loop of intestine is down in the hernial sac. This could cause a stoppage of intestinal function and death. A mare showing this condition or a stallion carrying this characteristic should not be used for breeding.

Cryptorchidism is a condition in which one or both testicles have not descended into the scrotum. Such stallions require major abdominal surgery for castration. Because this is an inherited condition and requires this kind of surgery for castration, it is not recommended that such stallions be used for breeding.

Lumbar myositis is manifested by tenderness over the back. The condition can be caused by a calcium-phosphorus imbalance, a poorly fitted saddle, higher vitamin-B requirements, soft tissue inflammation in the hind legs, and possibly other unknown factors. The tenderness can be so extensive as to interfere with the animal's use. If the animal responds to treatment, the unsoundness would only be temporary in nature. Unfortunately some animals seem to have a constant problem despite present treatment procedures.

COMMON BLEMISHES AND ABNORMAL CONDITIONS

The following conditions should not be considered unsoundnesses as they do not normally interfere with the utility of the animal.

Scars are only blemishes unless they mechanically interfere with normal activity of the horse.

Capped elbow is a soft tissue swelling over the point of the elbow (Fig. 29). It is a seroma (pocket of serum) that has resulted from the animal's injuring the area. This most often results from horses

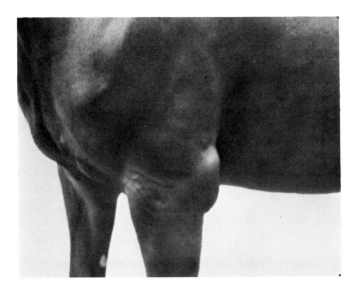

FIG. 29.   Capped elbow.

being bedded too lightly or not at all. As the animal attempts to get up from the hard floor or ground, the elbow comes in contact with the hard surface and the seroma results. The shoes may cause this injury when the animal is getting up.

Shoe boil is an infection over the point of the elbow. It may be the result of further injury to a capped elbow caused either by ground pressure or a shoe. The condition is treated as an open wound. Ample clean straw should be supplied for bedding.

Splints are bony enlargements (calcium deposits) usually located high on the inside of the front-leg cannon bones. They occasionally occur on the outside of the cannon bones and also on the hind legs. They are the result of the tearing of the small ligaments that hold the normal small splint bones to the cannon bone. This tearing causes a small hemorrhage into the area, where the blood clots and often turns into a calcium deposit. Splints rarely cause lameness. A few cause temporary soreness at the time of the initial tearing of the ligaments. Some large calcium deposits high on the inside of the cannon bone can encroach on the joint and cause lameness. Initial use of ice packs, rest, and aspirin is helpful. Local injections of corticosteroids directly into the developing deposit often stop further enlargement and stimulate some resorption. The author opposes the use of the firing iron for this condition or any other. DMSO is useful. Most all disappear in time.

Wind puffs are soft enlargements just above the fetlocks (Fig. 30). They are swellings from increased fluid in the tendon sheaths.

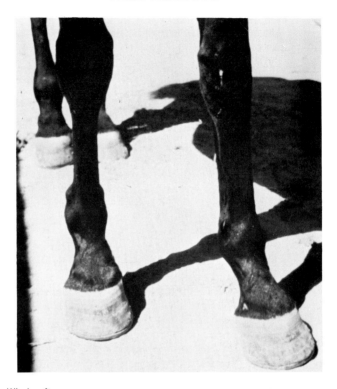

FIG. 30.   Wind puffs.

Long pasterns, letting the toe grow too long, and strenuous work on hard surfaces can predispose the horse to this condition. They rarely cause lameness except for those few that develop extreme internal pressure. These are usually the result of a sprain. Sometimes draining them and injecting cortisone into them helps, but they have a tendency to recur despite treatment. They only represent a blemish.

Bog spavin is a swelling of the hock joint capsule (Fig. 31). Though a straight-hock conformation may predispose to the condition, strain seems to be the most common cause. Characteristically, there are three swellings of the joint capsule. There is one on each side of the back area of the hock, and the third and largest swelling occurs on the inside forward aspect of the joint. The condition is most common in young horses up to 2 years old, but may occur in adults. It rarely causes lameness; so it is usually just a blemish. Draining, injection of corticosteroid drugs, and confined rest with or without bandaging often are effective treatments, though the condition has a tendency to recur. Bog spavins usually go away by themselves as the young horse continues to grow. The author strongly opposes entering any joint unless absolutely necessary.

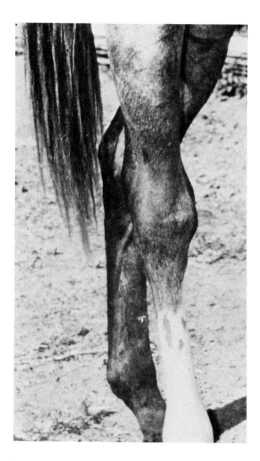

FIG. 31.   Bog spavin.

Bone spavin is a bony enlargement (calcium deposit) low on the inside of the hock. Poor hock conformation with excessive concussion can cause the condition. A temporary lameness often occurs at the onset of the development of the spavin. The horse can "warm out" of this lameness with a little exercise, but stiffness to the joint reappears after resting. The injection of corticosteroids directly over the enlargement with or without the initial use of ice packs and a 2- to 3-month rest period is often effective in allowing the spavin to "set," after which it no longer causes lameness. Rest alone may be effective, but surgery may be indicated for chronic cases of lameness. DMSO can be useful.

The *spavin test* is useful to help diagnose the condition. The affected leg is held up, tightly flexed against the body for a few minutes. The leg is then released and the horse is quickly trotted away from the examiner. The test is positive if the lameness is markedly accentuated for the first few steps after being released. A rope burn, a wound behind the pastern, or an injured fetlock may give a false-positive spavin test.

Thoroughpin is a soft swelling in the outside web of the hock. It rarely causes any problems and is usually just a blemish.

Curb is a bony enlargement on the back surface of the leg below the point of the hock and is the result of an inflammation to a ligament in that area. Sickle hocks predispose to this condition. Only a temporary lameness may occur with the onset of a curb. The condition is not considered serious.

Capped hocks (Fig. 32) are those that have a soft, flabby enlargement of the skin over the point of the hock. They result from a direct injury, such as results from kicking inside a trailer. The irritation causes an increase in the amount of fluid in the bursa

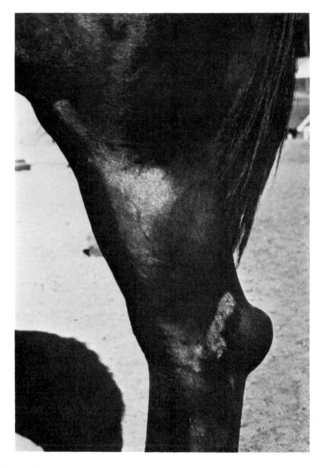

FIG. 32. Capped hock.

over the hock. Early cases are best treated with corticosteroids and draining if the fluid pocket is well established. Ice packs or cold water baths are helpful. DMSO is useful and effective.

After a few days, a fibrinous scar tissue develops in the area, which is very difficult to treat effectively. Such hocks cause no problem but can represent an unsightly blemish.

COMMON VICES

Though the seriousness of a specific vice varies, it does detract from the potential desirability of pleasure of owning a given animal. A very bad temperament should be classified as an unsoundness; it can definitely affect the horse's usability and can be dangerous to the rider.

Personality vices are those that reflect the specific temperament and attitude of the animal. They include the following: biting, kicking, striking, shying, rearing, head tossing, halter pulling, running away, and tail wringing. Some horses with personality vices are difficult to catch, difficult to pick up feet, difficult to load in a trailer, or are constantly prancing while under the saddle. All of these are characteristics of a bad temperament and such animals are often dangerous to own. Unfortunately, a horse's temperament is well established at birth if not before, and it is next to impossible to change it. Though patience can work wonders with many animals, most ill-tempered horses are not worth the effort. "Life is too short to fight horses."

Stable vices are those that a horse exhibits in a stable or around other horses. *Cribbing* involves a horse grabbing a fence or other solid object with its teeth and swallowing air. This can predispose the animal to improper digestion and to being a "hard keeper." A cribbing strap helps stop this. Harmful affects are seldom caused by this habit, but it does frequently disturb the owner. If a cribbing strap is used, it should not be placed on the horse so tight that it causes discomfort or interferes with breathing. Pain-inflicting devices to prevent this habit should not be used because they are inhumane and their use cannot be justified. *Wood chewing* is common and most often is the result of boredom. Bot fly larvae activity and improper nutrition might be factors. It is worth noting that the use of old tires to "pad" feed mangers can be potentially dangerous. If the horses eat part of these old tires, it can cause severe intestinal impactions. *Viciousness toward other horses* is a very serious vice because such horses may permanently injure other animals.

4

General Care

GROOMING

Regular grooming cleans the hair and lessens the probability of skin disease and parasites. It is a convenient time to examine the entire horse, looking for wounds, parasite eggs, or skin disorders. With practice, grooming can be done with speed and thoroughness. It is good to groom horses daily. Those that are worked or exercised should be groomed before leaving and immediately after returning to the stable. Horses out in pasture are not often groomed daily, but it is always wise to clean out their feet frequently.

The usual grooming procedure involves currying and brushing the horse's coat, brushing or combing the mane and tail, cleaning the eyes if necessary, wiping out the nostrils and the area under the tail, and *cleaning the feet*. Heated, wet, or sweating animals should be cooled out before being groomed. On return from work or exercise, grooming should be done immediately (i.e., as soon as the tack is wiped off and put away).

Remove the excess water or perspiration with a sweat scraper and rub the horse briskly with a drying cloth to partially dry the coat. It should then be blanketed and walked until it is cool, allowing only a couple of swallows of water every few minutes while it is still cooling out. It is always dangerous to give a hot horse free access to water.

Grooming Equipment

General grooming equipment consists of curry combs (rubber or metal), body brush, dandy brush, hoof pick, grooming cloth, drying cloth, safety razor, sweat scraper, and body sponge (Fig. 33).

Curry Comb

This is most commonly used to groom animals that have long, thick coats and to remove caked mud, loosen scurf and dirt in the hair, and remove loose hairs during shedding periods. It should be applied gently but firmly in small circles, and should never be used below the knees or hocks or about the head.

Body Brush

This is a fine, soft brush and is the principal tool for grooming. It can be used for brushing the entire body. Vigorous use not only removes dirt, but massages the skin and improves the luster of the coat.

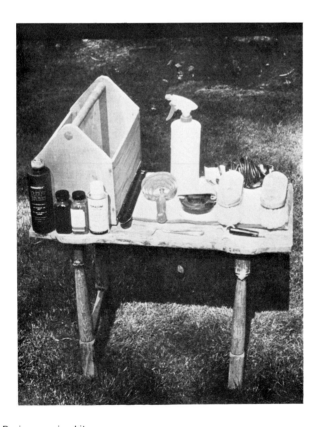

FIG. 33. Basic grooming kit.

Dandy Brush

This is a coarse brush and is used mainly on the lower legs to remove mud. It is also used for brushing the mane and tail, although hair conditioners are useful to take out the knots and prevent excess breaking of the hair when the mane and tail are to be kept as long as possible. A wire "poodle brush" or a large plastic comb often works well to brush out the mane and tail.

Hoof Pick

This should be the most frequently used piece of grooming equipment. Many commercial types are available, but if necessary, a screw driver or even a nail may be used. The important part of cleaning out the hoof is to thoroughly clean out the bottom of the depression between the frog and the bars, which is the usual site of thrush. Work from the heel toward the toe. A thorough washing with water of the undersurface of the hoof is advisable once a week. If the hooves become dry and crack or chip easily, they should also be painted, as needed, with a good hoof dressing, lanolin, or any other absorbable form of animal oil.

Grooming Cloth

This is used to remove dirt and dust from the tips of the hair, to wipe off the head, to clean the dock, and to generally polish the coat. Old blankets or towels cut into 2-foot squares serve this purpose.

Drying Cloth

This is used to dry perspiration or to massage the skin. Cut-up grain sacks or towels make good drying cloths. A compact handful of bedding or hay can be used as a substitute.

Safety Razor

This is used to remove bot eggs from hairs on legs, neck, and head.

Sweat Scraper

A flexible strip or a curved inflexible piece of metal is the best material for this useful tool. It is used to remove excess moisture from sweating or recently bathed animals. A lot of walking can be saved by the use of a sweat scraper.

Body Sponge

This is used for bathing horses, or applying certain insecticides, repellents, or hair conditioners. A wet body sponge is often routinely used for cleaning the face and dock.

Washing Grooming Equipment

Grooming equipment, as well as tack, should be frequently cleaned and disinfected as a precaution against skin diseases. It is best to have individual equipment for each horse. Amway's Germicidal, Nolvasan, or other good disinfectants that are also fungicidal should be used. To stiffen the bristles of brushes after disinfection, soak them for approximately 10 minutes in a concentrated salt solution (add salt to water until no more salt can be dissolved), and stand brushes with bristles down, to dry.

Grooming Methods

Grooming should be done in a routine manner. First, all four feet are thoroughly cleaned. Next, the body is well groomed, working from the neck backward. The head, mane, and tail are then brushed. Finally, with the grooming cloth, the face, eyes, nostrils, and dock are cleaned. A final polish is then given to the coat. If the weather is cool or if the animal is being prepared or maintained for show purposes, a horse blanket should be put on as soon as grooming is completed. It should be set down carefully so that it does not force the hairs in the wrong direction.

Pulling Manes and Tails

Individual hairs of a horse's mane and tail are often pulled out to make the mane and tail appear thin and even. This is usually done to conform to a particular breed's standard of appearance. This is done by grasping a few hairs at a time and sliding the hand up close to the roots, then giving a quick jerk. The longest hairs on the underside are worked first. Tails are often shortened to about four inches below the hocks. Scissors or clippers are never used to shape the tail, although sometimes the mane is clipped off, or "roached," as in the working quarter horse.

Cleaning the Sheath

The sheath is the skin that forms a pocket around and contains the penis (Fig. 34). It collects secretions and dead skin-surface cells, which are called smegma. This collection of material is foul-smelling and can build up inside the sheath and be a source of irritation to the horse. It is not uncommon for this fatty smegma to accumulate into a ball in the small blind pocket located just

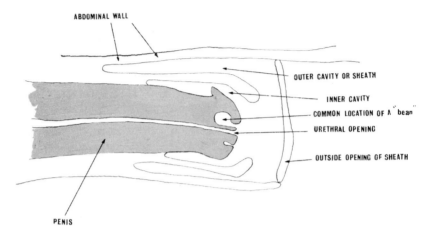

FIG. 34.   Anatomy of the sheath.

above the urethral opening in the end of the penis. The ball of smegma is called a "bean." Occasionally, this "bean" becomes so large that it interferes with normal urination.

Tail rubbing is a common symptom of a male horse that is irritated by a dirty sheath. All stallions and geldings should have their sheaths cleaned at least every 6 months and more often if necessary. A male horse with a white genital area, such as an Appaloosa or Pinto, has a tendency to accumulate smegma faster and should have its sheath cleaned more frequently.

The technique of cleaning the sheath is not difficult and most horses do not object if you proceed quietly and gently. For very nervous animals, a twitch is applied (see Chapter 6, under *Restraint*). The horse is put in a cross tie or is held next to a wall or fence so that it cannot move in circles. A helper should be available to steady the animal at the head, holding the lead rope close to the halter. It is best not to tie a nervous animal for this procedure.

The materials needed are a plastic bucket, warm water, a roll of cotton, and a mild soap such as L.O.C. or Ivory. Most mild liquid dish soaps are satisfactory as long as the area is well rinsed after the cleaning is finished. The procedure is as follows:

1. Place a fair amount of the cotton into a bucket of warm water.
2. Take a small handful of the wet cotton and apply the liquid soap to it (Fig. 35).
3. While quietly standing in close to the animal's left side, the soapy cotton is slowly carried up deep into the sheath (Figs. 36 and 37).
4. The whole area of the sheath and the penis is soaped and cleaned. As a piece of dirty cotton is brought out and disposed of, another soapy piece is used for further cleaning.

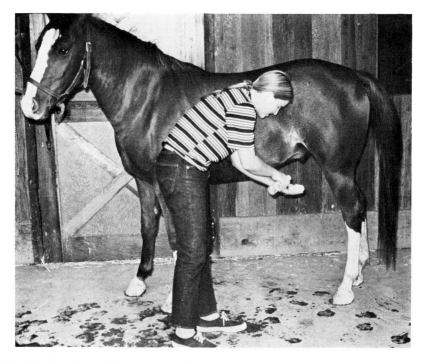

FIG. 35.   Soap is applied to wet cotton (Pat Schwarz).

The penis can be thoroughly cleaned within the sheath; it need not be forcibly pulled out of the sheath. While cleaning the penis, the blind pocket located just above the urethral opening in the end of the penis should be explored with the finger to detect and remove any "bean" that has built up (Fig. 38).

5. After all the smegma has been removed, fresh, nonsoapy wet cotton is used for thorough rinsing of the sheath. As much wet cotton as needed should be used to rinse all soap from the area. Soap residue can be irritating inside the sheath. On a warm day, with a gentle horse, a garden hose can be used for the rinsing.

It is a good practice to periodically examine the head of the penis carefully to note any possible tissue growth. Such tissue is often cancerous (a squamous cell carcinoma). Early detection and treatment are important because such a growth may necessitate amputation of the penis to avoid allowing the cancer to spread internally and cause death.

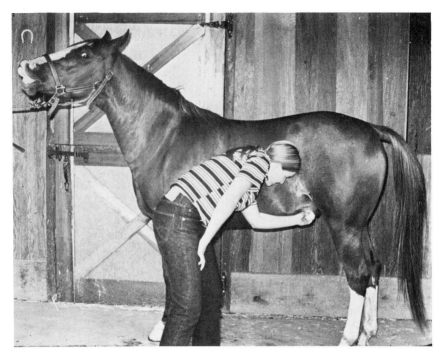

FIG. 36.   Soapy wet cotton is taken up into the sheath. Most horses don't really object.

WASHING

A thorough cleaning often requires a bath with soap and water to rid the coat of old sweat, scurf, and dirt. (Amway's L.O.C. soap is a good general soap for bathing horses.) Frequent, unnecessary bathing should be avoided in cool weather. Chilling lowers an animal's resistance to disease and often predisposes it to respiratory infections. Thorough drying of the wetted hair and skin to prevent chilling can be accomplished by removing the excess water with a sweat scraper and by vigorous use of a drying cloth. The horse is then walked with a cooler or blanket until dry.

BLANKETING

Blankets of various types are used for the following purposes:
1. As protection against cold and storm.
2. To cool out wet or heated animals.
3. To improve the coat for show purposes.
4. To protect sensitive animals from flies.
5. As a protection against chill in the case of sick animals.

Many types of blankets are commercially available, from light

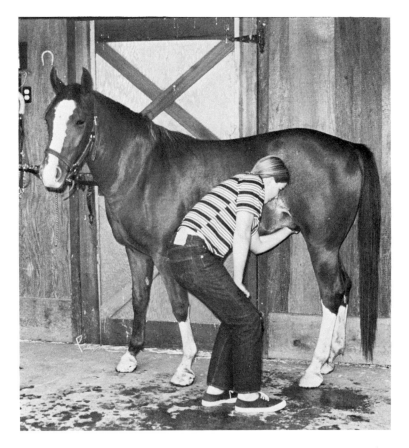

FIG. 37. The penis does not have to be brought out in order to thoroughly clean the sheath.

sheets to heavily lined blankets. Heavy horse blankets used on stabled horses in cold weather are desirable and appreciated.

A blanket should be properly adjusted and secured to prevent its slipping, otherwise frightening the animal, or becoming torn. It should be kept clean and in good repair. A blanket used on an animal suffering from a communicable disease should be thoroughly disinfected before it is used on another animal. It is best to have specific blankets for individual horses to prevent spread of skin disease and parasites. Sometimes it is necessary to cross-tie or put a "bib" on an animal that bites at its blanket. It may be dangerous to turn a horse out with a blanket on. A nonwaterproof blanket should not be used on a horse that is out in the rain.

CLIPPING

As a rule, clipping a horse or pony is not recommended unless it is heavily worked or is being prepared for a show. Whether

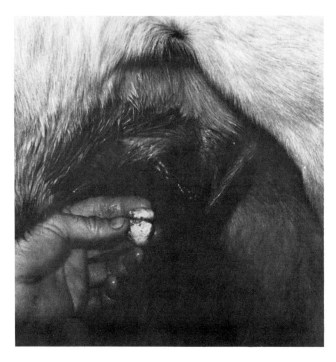

FIG. 38.   A "Bean" removed from the blind pocket in the end of the penis.

clipping is advisable depends on several factors, such as the nature of the coat, the climatic conditions, the amount and character of work to be performed by the animal, and the protection afforded by the stable facilities.

Clipping has the disadvantages of causing the horse discomfort in cool weather and lowering its resistance to disease. However, clipped animals that are heavily worked are less easily overheated, show more endurance, and require less time to cool out. (Clipping, however, should never be used as a substitute for good grooming!)

Where animals are to receive considerable work under saddle, it is advisable to leave an unclipped saddle patch the size of the saddle blanket. During cold weather, it is not advisable to clip the legs. Clipped animals should not be exposed to low temperatures in corrals or pastures, and should always be stalled and blanketed during the winter months. Heat lamps are also useful.

CARE OF THE FEET

The hoof is made up of three distinct outer structures: the *wall,* the *sole,* and the *frog.* The horse grows a completely new hoof every nine months. Because of this continuous growth, the wall gets long and needs to be trimmed. The thickness of the sole increases and normally has a whitish flaking as it grows out. The frog also grows out, gets broader, and needs regular trimming and shaping. If the frog is allowed to expand uncontrolled, it will cover the crevice or grooves that separate it from the sole, causing a moist condition deep in these crevices, which allows the development of *thrush* (Fig. 39). The routine trimming of the frog opens these crevices to air and preserves the normal conditions necessary for a healthy frog and foot.

The sole is not meant to be a weight-bearing structure. The weight of the horse is meant to be supported by the wall of the hoof. If a horse is to be left unshod, the sole should be hollowed in a concave manner to minimize any weight-bearing and the possibility of stone bruises.

Proper care of the feet should be one of the horseman's main considerations for the horse's well-being and to help assure the horse's usability. If the horse is kept shod, the shoes should be replaced or reset *every 4 to 6 weeks.* Horses, broodmares, and colts that are not shod should have their feet trimmed *at least every 8 weeks!* Even if a horse is not working, shoes should never be left on all winter. If they are allowed to stay on this long, the hooves become very long, causing excessive strain on the tendons and even lameness (Fig. 40). Also, prolonged standing in mud and moist conditions without frequent cleaning out of the feet can result in thrush. This condition can undermine the entire frog, resulting in a deep foot infection and lameness. Routine cleaning out of the feet and regular trimming of the hooves can help minimize this problem. Twice-a-week application of a drug preparation called Kopertox can help prevent the condition from occurring. This is true even in midwinter when the animals are out standing in moisture for weeks at a time. Kopertox has a non-water-soluble base and leaves a bandagelike coating.

The use of mud baths, oils, or hoof dressings is helpful in treating and preventing excessively *dry feet* in the summer. Allowing the water trough to overflow is a simple technique to see that the horses get access to some mud.

The feet of a foal should be trimmed beginning at the age of 1 or 2 months, at which time only a rasp is needed to shape the hoof. Early attention can help correct or prevent such leg problems as toeing in or toeing out. Abnormal leg and tendon problems should be brought to the attention of a veterinarian at an early stage of development.

The best indication of the health of a hoof is the condition of the frog. If the frog is excessively dry and hard or recessed, it indicates that it is not in proper contact with the ground and that,

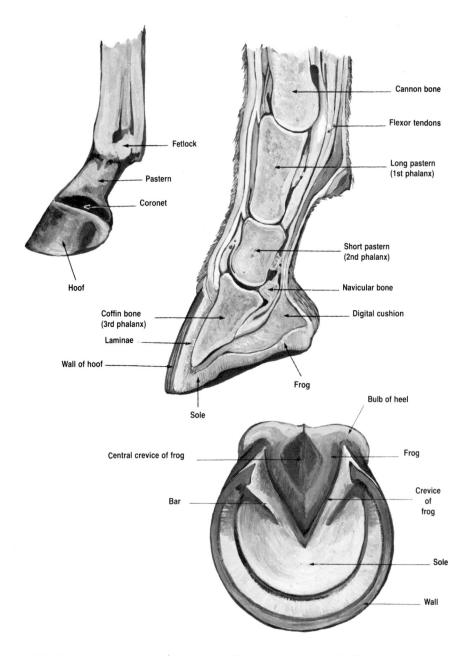

FIG. 39.   *A*, Structures of the leg and foot. (Drawings by Jeannine Quilici.)

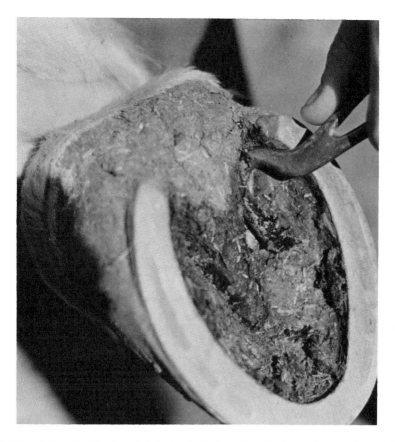

FIG. 39.   *B*, Thrush with characteristic black, foul-smelling discharge along crevices of the frog.

consequently, foot circulation is poor. This leads to excess drying of the hoof and dry, cracking walls. Poor shock-absorption ability of the hoof results. This, in turn, can cause the foot to sustain more jarring or rough concussion than it normally would, which predisposes the animal to such conditions as ringbone, sidebone, and navicular disease.

The keys to good, healthy feet are normal moisture and elasticity. The most important factor in hoof health is proper expansion and contraction. The feet should be trimmed and shod so that the feet hit the ground flat, straight, level, and in perfect balance—with *frog pressure*. The frog is important in stimulating normal blood circulation in the foot by coming into contact with the ground (thus creating a pumping action). Because of this, it

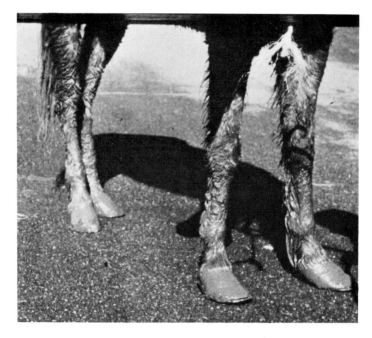

FIG. 40. Allowing the feet to grow too long can cause serious damage to the legs and feet, e.g., tendonitis, corns, deep thrush, and foot infections from "graveling."

is desirable to maintain a good, healthy frog by the frequent use of a hoof pick, proper trimming, and shoeing.[1]

Even the very best of shoeing is not good for the foot. If it is necessary, as it commonly is, to protect the foot or correct a gait or conformation fault, shoeing should be done with the lightest shoes possible, causing the least deviation from the normal axis and balance of the leg. Breeders who continually burden their poor horses with ungodly weighted shoes (Figs. 40A, B, C) create leg and foot problems and substantial excessive stress.

If horses are not trimmed and reshod at frequent, regular intervals, the result can be dry, contracted, unhealthy frogs, and thus potential foot problems.[2]

If a horse's hooves were trimmed every 2 weeks, it probably would never need shoes.

---

[1]When the wall of the hoof grows, it follows the shoe. If it is desired to reduce the width of a splayed or extra-broad hoof, a slightly reduced size shoe is used. If attempting to widen a heel or to enlarge a small hoof, a slightly larger than needed shoe is used.

[2]Eighty percent of lameness in the horse originates in the foot.

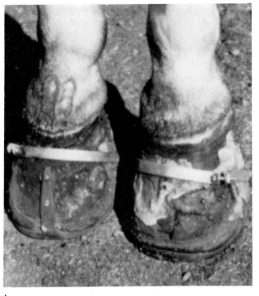

A

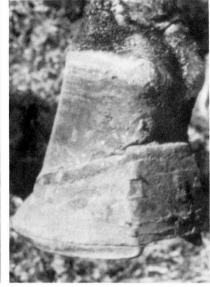

B

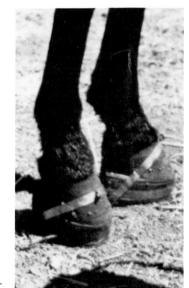

C

FIG. 40. *A, B, C.* Abnormally heavy shoes interfere with proper circulation to hooves and cause stress and excessive concussion to the feet and legs. They commonly cause pain and bony changes. They can rightfully be challenged from a humane concern.

Commonly Used Corrective Shoes

Bar Shoes with Pads

These shoes have a solid bar across the back, making a solid ring that is shaped to the foot. Under the shoes are pads (leather, padded plastic, or rubber). They are used in navicular disease to take pressure off the frogs and the painful back-third of the feet as well as in chronic laminitis during the recovery period to protect the very sensitive soles and to minimize painful foot contractions and expansions. Rolling of the toes allows the animal's steps to "break-over" faster, resulting in less jarring to the feet.

Normal Shoes with Full Pads or Rim Pads

Use: These shoes are used to treat bruised soles, to avoid excess concussion for beginning ringbone cases, to alleviate the hazards of sidebones, and to protect the feet of parade or taxi horses used on hard street surfaces.[3]

DENTAL CARE

A horse's teeth grow throughout its life. As was discussed earlier, it is because of this that the teeth can be used to determine the age of a horse because the teeth wear in a characteristic way. Though occasional problems arise from the irregular eruption of the front incisors, it is the back chewing teeth—the premolars and molars—that require routine care.

Wolf Teeth

The *wolf teeth* are small vestigial first premolars. These do not occur in all horses (Fig. 41). When they do occur, they appear just in front of the upper first chewing teeth—in either sex. It seems that horses are going through a process of evolution, doing away with these teeth much as man is doing away with wisdom teeth. Perhaps less than 40% of horses have these teeth. A horse may have two or just one. These teeth may be very small with a very small root and may be set just inside the gum, or they can be quite large with a well-developed root. Sometimes they do not erupt from the gum surface, but grow horizontally under the gums. It is the wolf teeth that grow under the gum and those that have very poorly developed roots that cause problems (Fig. 42).

Signs

Horses with sensitive wolf teeth are characteristically difficult to bit or are "head tossers" when wearing a bridle. These symptoms do not occur when a hackamore or halter is used.

---

[3]Constant use of pads can result in excessively soft or thin soles. They should not be used during the winter, when moisture and sometimes mud is captured under the pad and thrush develops. It is advisable to alternate full pads with rim pads for horses that need this special shoeing.

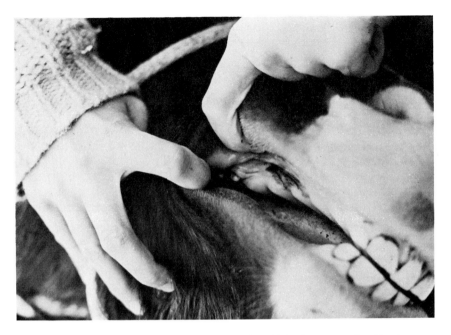

FIG. 41. Wolf tooth is a small vestigial first premolar which often causes head tossing.

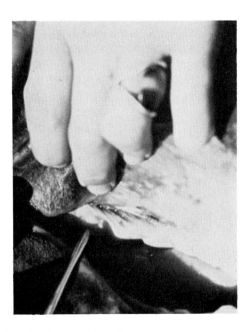

FIG. 42. Wolf tooth that didn't erupt from the gum, causing much pain when hit by a bit.

Procedure

If a horse has wolf teeth and is showing the characteristic signs, the wolf teeth should be removed. It is best to have this done under general anesthesia or sedation so that careful removal can be accomplished. Attempting to do this while the horse is standing is frequently dangerous to the veterinarian and may result in the breaking off of the root in the gum. This may cause a prolonged sore mouth and a long period of semi-dejection, less interest in eating, and the passage of small manure balls. With time, the animal gradually returns to normal, but may require veterinary attention. Normal extractions only leave the mouth sore for a few days, and the "head tossing" usually subsides within 2 weeks.

Sharp Dental Points

As the back chewing teeth continue to grow, the uppers and lowers wear in such a way that they cause sharp points to develop on the edges of the teeth. Since the uppers overlap the bottom teeth toward the outside, and the lowers overlap to the inside, wounds will occur to the inside cheek area and along the margin of the tongue. The pain caused by these points discourages the horse from chewing well and causes it to take a long time to eat. It is a common misbelief held by many horsemen that this is only a problem in aged horses. It is not uncommon that teeth need filing (floating) as early as age 18 months. The particular bite or inherited position of the teeth can influence how early or how often teeth need attention. A *wavy mouth* is a condition that may develop in older horses, but is sometimes seen in horses younger than 10. The chewing surfaces of the back molars wear irregularly, giving them a wavy top surface. Such teeth most often need attention every 6 months.

Signs

Slow eating and excessive mouthing of the feed with or without excessive salivation are common symptoms. Because horses, as well as other animals, have no digestive enzymes to digest away the outer layer of hay—a complex carbohydrate called lignin—they depend on good chewing to help in better utilization of the feed. Sharp dental points often attribute to a horse being a "poor keeper."

Procedure

The teeth should be examined routinely each year or as often as every 6 months for some horses, to determine whether there is any evidence of the development of these points. This examination is best done with the use of a metal dental wedge to allow a better examination of the back teeth with minimal danger to the examiner. Frequently, deep lacerations or grooves are observed inside the cheeks and along the tongue. The offending points are filed down with the use of dental rasps called "floats." This "floating" of the teeth can give great relief to affected horses and can markedly improve their feed utilization and reduce their eating time. Most horses will develop substantial points within 12 months.

Defective Molars and Premolars

These defects are common in older horses. Though horses rarely have "cavity" problems, diseased gum lines and abscessed roots are frequently found in aged horses, especially those over 20 years old.[4]

Signs

Difficult, prolonged chewing (often with *excessive salivation*), and a rotten odor on the breath are common signs. When the teeth are examined far back in the mouth, the faulty teeth are frequently out of alignment with the other teeth and the gum lines have receded from the roots. The teeth are also loose when handled. Such horses are usually very poor keepers and may be dull and sluggish and are prone to constipation and colic.

Procedure

Removal under a general anesthetic is indicated, followed by the use of antibiotics to clear up local mouth infections. On rare occasions, it is necessary to "punch out" a diseased tooth through a surgical opening in the sinus over the tooth. When many teeth have been lost, it is necessary to give such horses special diets, requiring less chewing, in order to retain good flesh and condition.

TRAILERING HORSES

Loading a horse into a trailer can often be a difficult procedure if that animal is not well trained or accustomed to it. Tranquilizers are often beneficial to a nervous animal. The following three techniques may be useful when handling a reluctant "loader":

---

[4]Routine dental care can add much to a horse's general state of health and well-being and should be part of a horse's routine medical care program. Though it is true that many horses in the wild do live long lives, their life expectancy is generally much less than that of our well-cared-for domestic horses and the latter enjoy a better state of general health.

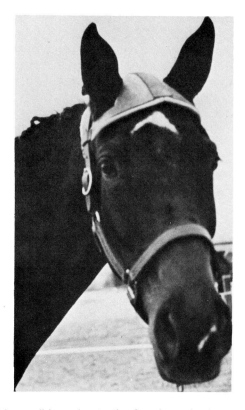

FIG. 43. A "head bumper" is good protection for a horse that has a tendency to rear in a covered trailer.

1. Coax it in with grain and close the tailgate behind it.
2. Place a long lead rope from the animal's halter into the tie-ring in the trailer and back out again to get his head in; tie a sideline to either side of the trailer to help guide the animal; then quietly bring this rope around behind the animal to direct it in. If it continues to back out, the third procedure may be tried.
3. Line the animal up as described in the second procedure. Since very few horses will kick at this point, it is often possible for two men to interlock their hands with an "Indian grip" behind the rump of the animal to force it in. This should be done cautiously. It is often possible to manually lift up its rear quarters to put it in, but this is best only attempted by an experienced horseman.

It is always best to drive evenly with smooth starts and stops when pulling an animal in a trailer. Avoid sharp and fast turns.

In general, it is good to rest animals after every 4 hours of trailering.

When trailering mares with very young foals, it is a good idea to have them separated by a full divider to prevent the foal from accidentally being stepped on by the mare. Shut the space above the tailgate door tightly to prevent the foal from attempting to jump out. Never tie young foals.

Always tie the horse securely in the trailer to a tie-ring at the feed stall area. Use the usual, easily untied slip knot as a safety measure in the event the animal falls down in the trailer.

Almost any animal can be made to go into a trailer after being treated by a veterinarian with the use of both tranquilizers and sedatives. Since horses can be "awakened" out of the effect of a tranquilizer, they frequently also need a sedative to stop them from their persistent reluctance to getting into the trailer. A proper dosage can be established by the attending veterinarian. The drug Rompum works very well for this purpose. After the use of this drug, any horse can be gotten into a trailor within 10 to 15 minutes (the author has seen no exceptions). It is also advisable to put a "head bumper" (a pad over the horse's poll) on reluctant horses that have a tendency to rear in the trailer (Fig. 43).

PART
II

Nutrition and Reproduction

CHAPTER

5

Equine Nutrition

The proper feeding of horses requires more knowledge, experience, and good judgment than with any other class of livestock. Unfortunately, horses are, in general, the most poorly fed (Figs. 44 and 45). This is mainly due to a great lack of information about equine nutrition on the part of both horse owners and nutritionists. Further research is needed to resolve many unanswered questions. Unfortunately, there is more to proper feeding than just throwing the horse some hay.

Basically, horses, like other animals, digest and utilize feed as proteins, carbohydrates, fats, vitamins, and minerals. The specific requirements for these nutrients depend on the amount of work or production demanded of the horse. From feeding trials and studies, mostly with other animals other than horses, specific requirements for horses have been calculated and recommended by the National Research Council in Washington, D.C.

In order to discuss nutrition in the horse, we must discuss common sources of nutrients for them. It then becomes necessary for us to have certain standards by which we can compare feeds to better understand their relative nutritional values. Although there are many ways of comparing feeds, this discussion is limited to the factors known as *total digestible nutrients, digestible protein, and calcium–phosphorus ratios,* which are the most important. This limitation may make the subject a little less confusing. The important physical characteristics of feeds, such as their being clean, palatable, free of mold, not too heavy or bulky, or too laxative, or too constipating, and the necessity for the overall ration to be balanced are also discussed here.

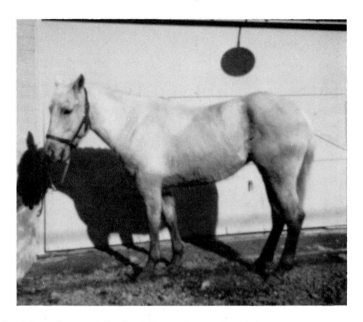

FIG. 44.   A horse in poor state of nutrition and general condition.

The *total digestible nutrients* (TDN) value of a feed represents the percentage of the feed that is digestible and usable by the animal. In general, feeds with high fiber content have low TDN values. Hays (roughages) are approximately 50% digestible and therefore have a TDN of 50%. Grains (concentrates) have less fiber, are about 75% digestible, and have a TDN of approximately 75%. Poor curing and poor storage can lower the TDN values of feed.

The *digestible protein* (Dig. Prot.) values are also important because proteins are important building blocks for body cells. In general, the greater the Dig. Prot. is, the greater is the overall feed value (and its cost). When feeds are chemically analyzed, *crude protein* figures are given. These also represent some non-protein compounds. Because of this, the crude protein values of a feed are higher than their true Dig. Prot. value. The Dig. Prot. for grains (concentrates) is approximately 80% of the crude protein value. Therefore, the Dig. Prot. of a grain can easily be calculated. For example, oats have a crude protein value of 9% and this figure multiplied by 0.8 (80%) equals 7.2%. Dig. Prot. Actually, the Dig. Prot. for oats is considered to be 7.0%. The Dig. Prot. of hays (roughages) is about 60% of the crude protein value. For example, oat hay crude protein is 8.2%. This multiplied by 0.6 (60%) equals 4.92%. The known Dig. Prot. value for oat hay is 4.9%. This relationship is more variable with hays than with grains.

The *calcium–phosphorus ratio* (Ca:P) is a very important concern

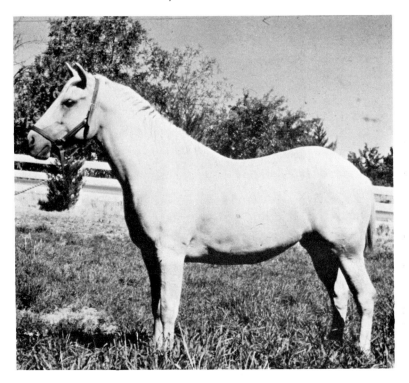

FIG. 45. The same horse after being wormed, having the teeth floated, and being put on a good feeding program for 4 weeks.

when feeding horses. It represents the relative intake of calcium to that of phosphorus. Ideally, the Ca:P ratio for a horse's overall daily ration should be 1:1 or 2:1. Every 1 part or 2 parts calcium taken in should be accompanied by 1 part phosphorus. When the Ca:P is unbalanced, many muscle and bone problems can occur. Most frequently, problems occur from excess phosphorus rather than from too much calcium, such as ratios of 1:5 or 1:6 and occasionally when the ratio is as close as 1:1.4. The author has not experienced problems from excess calcium in the diet.

QUICK RUN-DOWN ON SOME COMMON FEEDS

Roughages

Alfalfa Hay

It is economical and entirely safe when fed properly (Fig. 46). It can be fed as the only hay, which is being done by many breeding farms. If it is cut before full bloom, it is often laxative. It stimulates body metabolism and is highly palatable, though

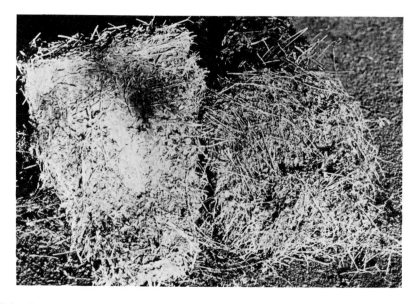

FIG. 46. Not all alfalfa is good quality. If allowed to leach, bleach, or mold, its value is markedly reduced. Moldy hay is always potentially dangerous to horses.

overeating on hay (roughage) is never a problem. Alfalfa is good for growth and milk production and is high in vitamins A, D, B_2, and niacin. It has good-quality protein and is recommended to constitute at least one-half of the hay ration to make up for other hay deficiencies.

TDN	Dig. Prot.	Ca:P
50.3	10.5	7:1

Oat Hay

Oat hay is satisfactory as the only hay for mature idle horses. However, it is low in protein and it is best to give a protein supplement in addition. It is also low in calcium. It is important that oat hay be cut and cured properly, retaining some color and lots of grain. For any type of production, or for young growing stock, additional supplements are necessary.

TDN	Dig. Prot.	Ca:P
47.3	4.9	1:1

Timothy Hay

This hay's popularity is due to the ease with which it can be grown and cured into bright hay that is free from dust and mold. It is low in protein, but fine for mature, working stock if it is properly supplemented. It is definitely not sufficient for production of milk or growing foals.

TDN	Dig. Prot.	Ca:P
48.9	2.9	1:1

Barley Hay

This hay is somewhat similar to oat hay in value except that it is lower in protein and often causes mouth wounds.

TDN	Dig. Prot.	Ca:P
51.9	4.0	1:1

Volunteer Hay

Volunteer hay is usually low in protein and has a high fiber content, thus it is a poor overall feed. It is often a cause of many mouth wounds, abscesses, and irritation from foxtails. Volunteer hay is not recommended as a standard ration for horses, especially if working or in production. Hay with foxtails and bearded barley should not be fed to horses (Figs. 47, 48, 49, and 50).

TDN	Dig. Prot.	Ca:P
46.7	.6	3:1

Green Pasture

Good green grass seems to have something quite superior in nutritive value. Horses on good, lush pasture come into full bloom, and put on weight. Good pasture is unexcelled by any other roughage in vitamin content, as well as palatability. Usually green pasture has around 15% TDN; however, as pasture grasses mature, the vitamin content as well as the palatability decreases. Young pasture is also much higher in protein and is more digestible. Pastures should be rotated, if possible, in order to avoid parasite problems. Hypothyroid horses should be kept off of green pastures to avoid foundering.

TDN	Dig. Prot.	Ca:P
14.9	3.7	2:1

See Figure 51 for a diagram of the seasonal trends in nutritional content of forage.

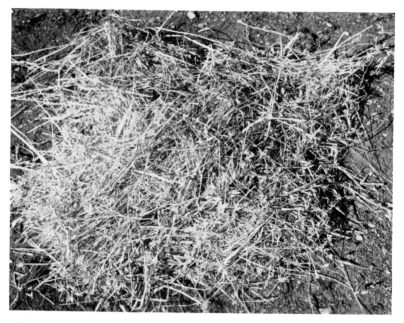

FIG. 47.　Poor-quality volunteer hay. It usually has very low nutritional value and frequently has many foxtails, which damage the mouths of horses.

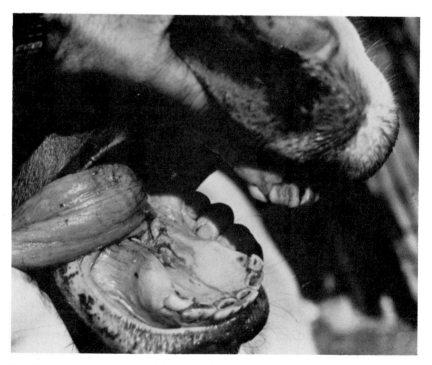

FIG. 48.　Mouths wounds caused by foxtails in poor-quality hay.

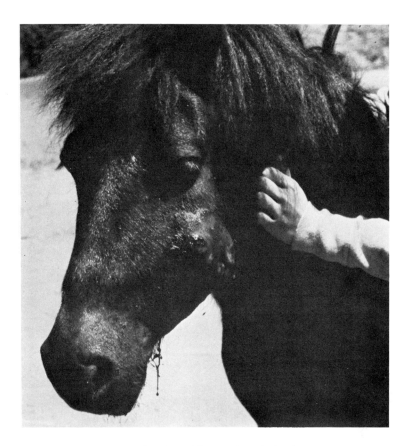

FIG. 49. Infections caused by foxtails working out through the tissues.

Concentrates

Oats, Rolled or Crimped

The Dig. Prot. of rolled or crimped oats is high enough to balance the deficiencies in grass hays. It has a relatively low TDN, however. Oats are the safest of all grains, and are the standard for horses. Grain rations of only oats, barley, corn barley, and bran, or mixtures thereof have Ca:P imbalances. A source of additional calcium, such as alfalfa hay, is needed.

TDN	Dig. Prot.	Ca:P
72.2	7.0	1:3

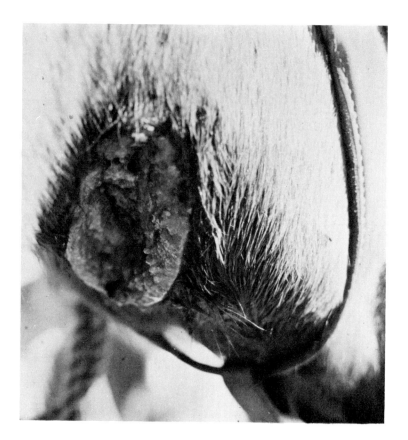

FIG. 50.   Infections caused by foxtails working out through the tissues.

Barley, Rolled

Rolled barley has good TDN but is low in protein. Horses do not chew *whole* barley well. Barley is much heavier than oats, and for this reason can cause colic if it is not mixed with bulkier feeds, such as oats. Nutritionally, it is about equal to oats, but higher in phosphorus.

TDN	Dig. Prot.	Ca:P
78.7	6.9	1:6

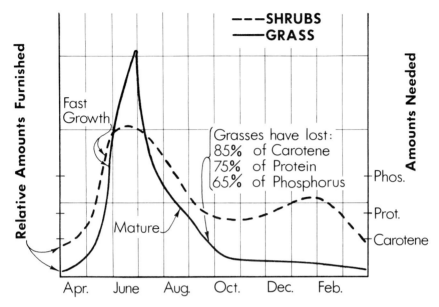

FIG. 51.   Seasonal trends in protein, phosphorus, and carotene content of range forage.

Corn, Cracked

Cracked corn is very palatable and high in vitamin A and fat and low in protein and calcium (only 0.4 pound of calcium in a ton). It is heavy and highly concentrated. Feed larger quantities with care. Corn has 15% less nutritional value than oats for working horses.

TDN	Dig. Prot.	Ca:P
80.1	6.6	1:13

Wheat Bran

Wheat bran is mostly the outer coatings of the wheat kernel. Bran is highly palatable and is mildly laxative. It is twice as bulky as oats and high in fat. It is also very high in phosphorus and has been associated with equine urinary calculi (bladder stones). It can be an important cause of Ca:P imbalance.

TDN	Dig. Prot.	Ca:P
67.2	13.7	1:9

Linseed Meal

Linseed meal is very palatable and slightly laxative. It has a conditioning effect. Horses on linseed meal shed out earlier and become sleek. It is an excellent protein source and good to give when using poor-quality hay. Don't use more than 1 to 1½ pounds per day, or 1 part to 16 parts corn and oats. The occurrence of temporary urticaria ("feed bumps") is not uncommon when using linseed meal. It is sometimes too laxative for some horses.

TDN	Dig. Prot.	Ca:P
77.2	30.8	1:3

Cotton Seed Meal

This meal is very high in phosphorus. It lacks vitamins A and D (like other seed products), but is fair in content of vitamin B. It produces hard fat and is slightly constipating. This meal is heavy and, in excess, can cause colic. It is possible to feed 1 to 1½ pounds per day, but ¼ pound per day is safe. It is very good-quality protein and produces good bloom.

TDN	Dig. Prot.	Ca:P
78.4	36.4	1:4

Soy Bean Meal

Soy bean meal is one of the best protein supplements. Soy bean meal has no vitamins A or D, but has sufficient quantities of vitamin B_1 and niacin. Feed no more than 1 pound per day; it is heavy and should be no more than one-third of the total mix. It has less phosphorus than cotton seed meal, linseed meal, and bran. It produces good bloom.

TDN	Dig. Prot.	Ca:P
78.6	37.5	1:2

Beet Pulp

Beet pulp is high in fiber but is well digested. It is high in calcium, but low in phosphorus. It lacks vitamins A and D but is bulky and fairly palatable. It is high in carbohydrates and energy, but relatively low in protein. It is often used to balance Ca:P ratios.

TDN	Dig. Prot.	Ca:P
67.8	4.3	6:1

Molasses

Molasses is a common supplement for horses. It adds value by increasing the palatability of other feeds, therefore cutting down on waste. Feed a maximum of 1 to 2 pounds per day. Amounts above this can be too laxative and can also cause increased sweating and inability to do heavy work during the summer. It is a good source of carbohydrates, iron, and calcium.

TDN	Dig. Prot.	Ca:P
54.0	0	9:1

Alfalfa Meal and Molasses

Alfalfa meal and molasses, nutritionally, is not much better than alfalfa hay alone, but may stimulate young stock to eat more and may be a good supplement for older horses with poor teeth. It is a good source of iron and energy and an excellent feed supplement when trying to put weight on an animal. It can be fed free-choice without danger of causing colic.

TDN	Dig. Prot.	Ca:P
50.6	9.0	4:1

Brewer's Yeast

This is an excellent source of vitamin B complex. It can equal linseed meal as a source of protein but is very high in phosphorus. The protein in it is one of the better plant proteins and seems to have a tonic effect from some unknown factor it contains. Two tablespoonfuls per day is an effective amount. Four tablespoonfuls per day can sometimes work miracles in calming nervous horses and helps ward off biting insects and external parasites.

TDN	Dig. Prot.	Ca:P
70.5	47.4	1:6

Salt

Salt is low in feeds of plant origin. A horse needs at least 2 ounces per day or 1 pound per week, depending on the weather and the amount of work the animal performs. Deficiencies can easily develop, causing poor growth, abnormal craving (such as is shown by fence chewers), stiff muscles, rough hair coat, and increased susceptibility to heat stroke. Allow free-choice trace mineral (red) salt blocks. Do not force feed.

VITAMINS

Vitamins are organic chemicals that are required for normal body functions. Deficiencies can cause failure to grow, reproduce, and maintain good health. Subclinical vitamin deficiencies cause the greatest economic loss due to their lack of obvious symptoms.

In the horse, we most frequently observe symptoms of vitamin A and B-complex deficiencies, although many other vitamins are also essential in the diet.

Deficiencies often occur under the following conditions: prolonged storage of feeds; low-quality feeds; forced and prolonged feeding; extended periods of drought; and excessive parasitism and dental problems.

Vitamin A

Vitamin A, clinically, is probably the most commonly deficient vitamin in the horse's ration.

Functions

1. Health of all epithelial tissue, such as the tissue lining the digestive, respiratory, and reproductive tracts, as well as the tissues of the skin and the cornea of the eye.
2. Growth of bones. (Poor bone growth can result in pressure on nerves, which can cause lack of coordination, spasms, and lameness.)
3. Prevention of night blindness.

Signs

The most obvious signs are those that affect the skin and hair coat (Fig. 52). The skin becomes very dry and scurfy. Black horses often take on a brown sunburned appearance. Palominos frequently become very pale. Runny eyes may be a symptom (Fig. 53). Hooves may become very dry and scaly (Fig. 53A). There is also a lowered resistance to respiratory infections, stress, and diarrhea.

Poor growth, knuckling of the fetlock, enlarged joints, and weak and crooked legs can be seen in foals (Fig. 54). Breeding animals may become less fertile.

Discussion

Green pasture and legume hays are probably the best natural sources of vitamin A. Vitamin A oxidizes rapidly in the air. Even when hay is well stored in a good barn, 80% is lost in 6 months. If hay heats or molds badly in curing or in storage, practically all the vitamin A is lost.

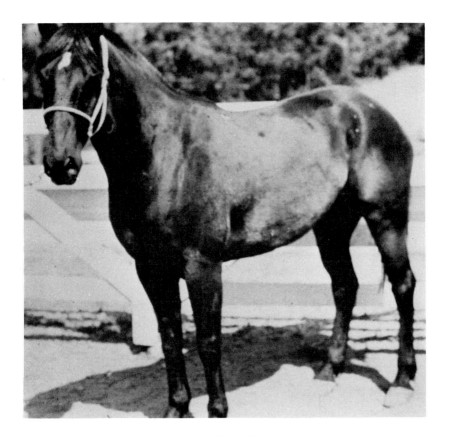

FIG. 52. Sunbleached coat from a vitamin A deficiency.

Because young animals are born with poor vitamin A storage and because deficiencies occur so frequently, it is good husbandry to supply a vitamin A supplement, especially to pregnant mares and growing colts. An "aqueous" form of vitamin A can be injected to give liver storage in 24 hours, whereas a prolonged vitamin A-deficient diet may require several months of tremendous oral supplements to produce liver storage.

Vitamin B Complex

Vitamin B-complex deficiencies are not uncommon in horses and can predispose the animal to a variety of symptoms.

Functions

These vitamins are involved with the coenzymes of carbohydrate, protein, and fat metabolism. The health and function of nervous tissue is dependent on the vitamin B complex, especially

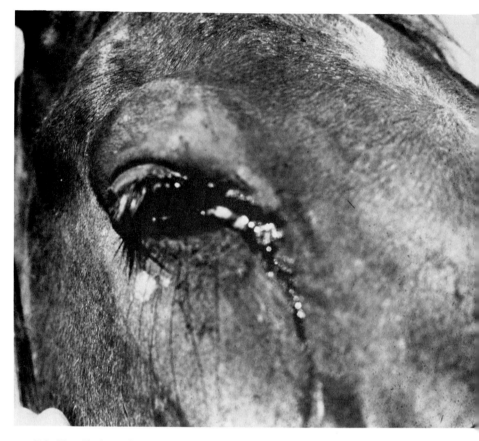

FIG. 53.   Discharge from eye secondary to vitamin A deficiency.

vitamin B$_1$ (thiamin). Growth, appetite, blood cell formation, and general well-being are adversely affected by deficiencies.

It appears that horses frequently manifest a greater vitamin B requirement during the winter cold months and when in training. Stress causes the body to use up more energy, which is derived from carbohydrate, protein, and fat metabolism, thus utilizing more vitamin B.

Signs

Excess nervousness, irritability, increased skin sensitivity, and leg edema are common signs. Tenderness over the back and dragging of the hind feet are frequently observed which may also be tied into Ca:P imbalances. Poor appetite, anemia, and wasting are other symptoms.

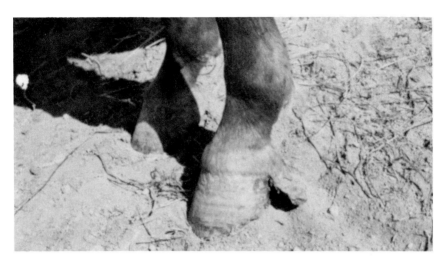

FIG. 53A. Vitamin A deficiency commonly causes dry hooves that crack easily. The photograph shows a torn quarter.

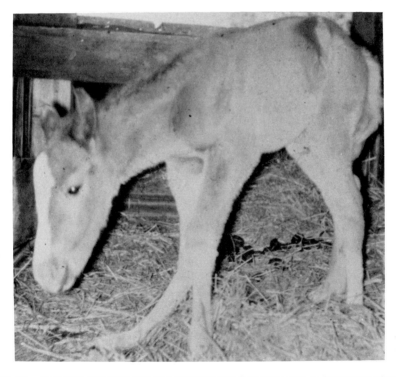

FIG. 54. Foal born with weak legs and poor hair coat from mare with an inadequate vitamin A intake during her pregnancy.

Prevention and Treatment

Good green pastures and legume hays are natural sources, but Brewer's yeast offers a very good vitamin B-complex supplement. Four tablespoonfuls per day are given the first week and then the dosage is reduced to two tablespoonfuls per day. This Brewer's yeast supplement is continued as long as it is necessary to prevent symptoms of vitamin B deficiency. It also appears to be valuable in making horses less "tasty" to biting insects, ticks, and lice.

Vitamin D

Vitamin D is very important in helping calcium to be absorbed from the gastrointestinal tract. Deficiencies result in bone weakness and rickets. Sunlight and alfalfa hay are both excellent sources. Race horses and other horses kept in stalls for prolonged periods of time with no access to sunlight are most affected. Excessive supplements of vitamin D should be avoided because too much can be toxic and may cause abnormal deposits of calcium in soft tissues or on bone, which could be an underlying cause for conditions like ringbone, sidebones, and spavins.

Vitamin E

Vitamin E, which was discovered in 1922, has gone through much debate about its value and its need as a dietary supplement. Because its supplementary use has not been clearly substantiated to have value in any area of equine activity (including reproduction) and because the author has not himself been convinced of its therapeutic effect in equine disease conditions, no specific recommendations are made here for its use or supplementation. This situation may change in the future as we come to know more.

Vitamin Supplements

In the general discussion on vitamins, it was pointed out that the most important vitamin deficiencies in the horse are of vitamins A and B-complex. This is not to say that the other known vitamins are not important to the horse, but it is not certain that their deficiency is a problem. Despite the large number of commercial vitamin preparations on the market for horses, the author knows of no single product that contains high contents of all particular vitamins to be used for therapeutic and maintenance levels. Most often, when supplements of the vitamin B complex are desired, Brewer's yeast should be given. When purchasing a general vitamin preparation, special attention should be given to what the vitamin A content per 1 pound is. Other products should be compared on the basis of cost of vitamin A per pound and the reliability of the manufacturer. Having additional multivitamins can offer "nutritional insurance."

MINERALS

Minerals are inorganic elements that play important roles in body chemistry. They are essential in the makeup of the skeleton, teeth, and blood cells. They are necessary constituents of many complicated biochemical activities of the normal metabolism of the body. Minerals play an important role in the fluid balance of body tissues and in the circulation of oxygen in the blood stream. Also, they are essential for blood cell formation, normal thyroid activity, and muscle metabolism. Of the fourteen known essential minerals, only nine are of practical concern in horses: calcium, phosphorus, sodium, chloride, iodine, cobalt, copper, iron, and magnesium. Deficiency of iron and magnesium can be a problem in suckling foals.

Signs

The effects of mineral deficiencies are usually subclinical and are not recognized or attributed to specific mineral deficiencies. Abnormal conditions such as rickets and osteomalacia are associated with Ca:P imbalances. Calcium deficiency is rare in the horse, but hays grown in phosphorus-deficient soils may not supply enough phosphorus for normal body activities. Almost any grain supplement program would prevent this from occurring. A long, continued *phosphorus deficiency* can cause stiffness of joints, fragile bones, abortions, weak foals, reduced fertility, reduced appetite, and decreased digestion efficiency.

Salt deficiencies can cause fatigue, unthriftiness, rough coats, loss of weight and production, dull eyes, weak foals, and pica (the abnormal hunger for unusual material such as wood, dirt, or manure). Secondary digestive upsets can occur. Wood chewing is also associated with boredom and mouth irritation from bot larvae migration in the tissues of the cheeks and tongue. These signs often disappear rapidly when salt is made available. A horse usually requires 2 to 3 ounces of salt daily. The higher amount is needed during the hot months. As a rule, it is best to have salt always available to the horse. Though some salt can increase feed palatability, too much can reduce it. Loose salt for horses is desirable, but salt blocks are satisfactory. Trace mineral salt blocks are available but are only necessary in areas known to have mineral-deficient soils. A horse owner should check with a local veterinarian or farm advisor for specific recommendations.

Commercial Mineral Supplements

It has become popular in some areas to feed highly advertised mineral or vitamin-mineral supplements. Not too long ago, many mineral mixes marketed for livestock were badly unbalanced and caused a great many problems by themselves, but more modern information has corrected most of these situations. Though vitamin supplements are definitely recommended, mineral supplements, other than a balanced source of Ca:P when needed, and a trace mineral salt block, are most likely unnecessary except in problem areas. It should be noted that many labels for commercial mixes often have long lists of chemicals and various ingredients that are most often included just to impress the prospective buyer. In the business, they are known as "eye wash." Again, check with a local veterinarian or farm advisor for specific recommendations. Iron supplements with vitamin B_{12} and the other B-complex vitamins are often given to horses in heavy training for their "blood building" value. Such products are often valuable.

FEATURES OF SOME COMMON FEEDS

High-Energy Feeds

These feeds (flaxseed meal, linseed meal, alfalfa meal, corn, molasses) are of special value during cold weather and for putting on weight. They are not recommended in large quantities for hard-working horses.

Protein Supplements

These feeds (cotton seed meal, linseed meal, soybean meal) are needed for growth, milk production, and to balance rations with poor-quality hays.

Heavy Feeds

Too heavy a grain ration can cause digestive problems. Heavy feeds are best fed along with bulkier feeds. Corn, barley, cotton seed meal, linseed meal, and soy bean meal are heavy feeds.

Bulky Feeds

These are helpful to use with heavy concentrates. Oats, beet pulp, and roughages are bulky feeds.

Laxative Feeds

Laxative feeds are helpful for mares heavy in foal, shortly after foaling, mild constipation, and for horses prone to impactions. Bran, linseed meal, molasses, and sometimes alfalfa are laxative feeds.

Constipating Feeds

These may be helpful for those horses prone to having loose manure. Cotton seed meal, and sometimes oat hay, has a constipating effect.

Feeds with Ca:P Imbalances

Commonly used feeds with Ca:P imbalances are oats, 1:3 (can be important); barley, 1:6 (can be important); corn, 1:13 (low in both, not likely to be important); bran, 1:9 (can be very important if much is being used); cotton seed meal, 1:4 (can be very important because it contains much phosphorus).

Calcium Sources

These are usually needed to offset high phosphorus intake in heavy graining schedules. The Ca:P of various calcium sources is alfalfa hay, 7:1; beet pulp, 6:1; molasses, 9:1; bone meal, 2:1; and shell flour, 2:1.

Good Vitamin Sources

Good sources of vitamins A and B complex are corn, carrots, alfalfa hay, green pastures (Vitamin A), Brewer's yeast, green pastures and grains (Vitamin B complex). It is best to supplement the diet with commercial preparations to ensure adequate intake of these vitamins.

COMPARING COMMERCIAL FEEDS

It has become popular to purchase ready-made or mixed commercial feeds. Since the exact formulas are not revealed, the owner has only the feed label by which to judge their relative values. One has to have faith in the companies that the feeds are nutritionally balanced. The labels must contain the contents of crude protein, crude fat, crude fiber, ash, and minerals.

It is the *crude protein* value that is the best indication of a feed's relative value. It is cost per pound that should be used to determine if a feed is a good buy or not. It should be emphasized that moldy, defective grain and moldy or weedy hay that may contain foxtail are never good buys at any price.

Feeds with a crude fiber value of 25% or more are roughages and should be compared to other roughages to determine their relative values on a crude-protein-per-pound basis. Feeds with a crude fiber value of 10% or less are concentrates. Tables I and II show comparisons among several feeds.

Comparing Vitamin Mixtures

Since almost all commercial vitamin mixtures for horses are not good supplements for the B complex, their relative values are best based on their vitamin A content (Table III).

It can readily be seen from Table III that Mixture 4 is by far the best purchase based on vitamin A content.

Horse Feed Requirements

A ration is the total daily intake of feed. The National Research Council (NRC) has established the nutritional requirements of the horse for different degrees of activity. The requirements change depending on what additional nutrients are required for the body to carry on the activities demanded of it. It is very important that all the nutritional needs be met in order not to cause a loss of conditioning or possible abnormality. If all these requirements are met, the ration is considered to be a *balanced ration* (Figs. 55, 56, and 57).

Table V is a chart of important nutritional requirements for a 1000-pound horse.

Computing a Ration

As can be seen, horses used for different purposes require different amounts and quality of nutrients (Figs. 55, 56, 57). By using

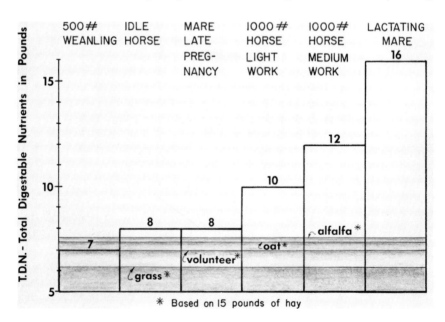

FIG. 55.   Equine nutritional requirement for T.D.N.

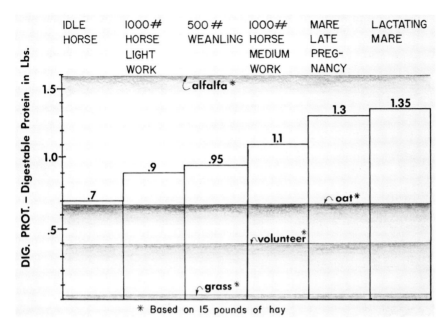

FIG. 56. Equine nutritional requirement for Dig. Prot.

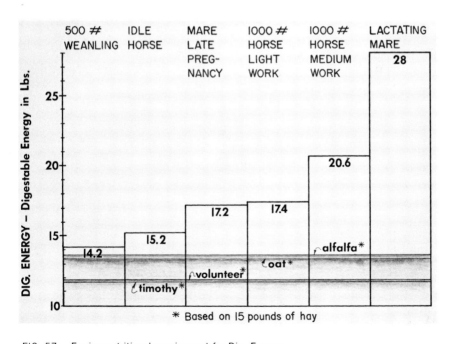

FIG. 57. Equine nutritional requirement for Dig. Energy.

(1) the "Requirements" chart (Table V) based upon the recommendations of the National Research Council, (2) the "Guidelines" chart (Table XI) which reflects those requirements, and (3) the "Feed Values" chart (Table IV), it is possible to calculate with fair accuracy the nutritional value of a given ration, and to create a ration by trial and error to meet the needs of horses used for various activities.

Example

Using the tables, we can determine the ration for a 1000-pound, mature, idle horse. Referring to Table XI, we see such a horse should only require about 15 pounds of good hay. Referring to Table V, we find that the figures are: TDN 7–9, Dig. Prot. 0.6–0.8, DM 13–18, Ca 0.033, and P 0.033 (Ca:P 1:1).

Let us see if just 15 pounds of oat hay will meet these requirements.

We can see that this ration may be just a little light on TDN and phosphorus, but not likely to be significant. If the hay were of very poor quality, then additional supplements would be necessary.

The method of computation is as follows: Since feed values are in percent, they are changed to their decimal form (e.g., TDN 50.3% = 0.503). This decimal figure multiplied by the amount of feed used (in pounds) equals the amount of nutrient in the feed.

If we were to give a ration of one-half alfalfa hay and one-half oat hay, the computation would be as follows.

CALCIUM-PHOSPHORUS IMBALANCES

Some of the most commonly recognized nutritional disorders are those due to a Ca:P imbalance. The ratio of the intake of calcium to the intake of phosphorus is especially critical in the horse. Ideally, this ratio should be 1 part or 2 parts calcium to 1 part phosphorus (e.g., 1:1 or 2:1). Most problems seem to occur when there is an excess of phosphorus as opposed to an excess of calcium. Studies have indicated that clinical problems can occur when the imbalance is as close as 1:1.4 and that of 1:1.6 causes problems to occur rapidly. Although horses can well tolerate a high-level intake of calcium with a wide Ca:P of 4:1 or more, high total quantity levels of *both* calcium and phosphorus can be harmful. A high-level intake of both calcium and phosphorus in one study of pregnant mares resulted in an increased rate of abortion, reduced birth weights of foals, and an increased incidence of abnormal bone developments in the foals.

Feed values of oat hay: TDN 46.3, Dig. Prot. 4.5, DM 88.1, Ca 0.22, P 0.17.						
Requirements	TDN	Dig. Prot.	DM	Ca	P	Ca:P
	7–9	0.6–0.8	13–18	0.033	0.033	1:1
Amount in pounds Feed						
15 Oat hay	6.9	0.68	13.2	0.033	0.026	1.3:1

TDN 0.463 × 15 = 6.945
TDN = 6.9

Dig. Prot. 0.045 × 15 = 0.675
Dig. Prot. = 0.68

DM 0.881 × 15 = 13.215
DM = 13.2

Ca 0.0022 × 15 = 0.0330
Ca = 0.033

P 0.0017 × 15 = 0.0255
P = 0.026

Ca:P 0.033 ÷ 0.026 = 1.2692
Ca:P = 1.3:1

Alfalfa hay—TDN 50.3, Dig. Prot. 10.6, DM 90.5, Ca 1.43, P 0.21
Oat hay—TDN 46.3, Dig. Prot. 4.5, DM 88.1, Ca 0.22, P 0.17

Requirements	TDN	Dig. Prot.	DM	Ca	P	Ca:P
	7–9	0.6–0.8	13–18	0.033	0.033	1:1
Amount in pounds Feed						
7½ Alfalfa hay	3.8	0.90	6.8	0.107	0.016	6.7:1
7½ Oat hay	3.5	0.34	6.6	0.017	0.013	1.3:1
15 lb. Total	7.3	1.24	13.4	0.124	0.029	4.3:1

Alfalfa Hay	*Oat Hay*
TDN 0.503 × 7.5 = 3.7725 TDN = 3.8	TDN 0.463 × 7.5 = 3.4725 TDN = 3.5
Dig. Prot. 0.106 × 7.5 = 0.7950 Dig. Prot. = 0.80	Dig. Prot. 0.045 × 7.5 = 0.3375 Dig. Prot. = 0.34
DM 0.905 × 7.5 = 6.7875 DM = 6.8	DM 0.881 × 7.5 = 6.6075 DM = 6.6
Ca 0.0143 × 7.5 = 0.10725 Ca = 0.107	Ca 0.0022 × 7.5 = 0.01650 Ca = 0.017
P 0.0021 × 7.5 = 0.01575 P = 0.016	P 0.0017 × 7.5 = 0.01275 P = 0.013
Ca:P 0.107 ÷ 0.016 = 6.6875 Ca:P = 6.7:1	Ca:P 0.017 ÷ 0.013 = 1.3077 Ca:P = 1.3:1

Signs

Bone Changes. Foals are especially affected because 90% of their bone skeleton is composed of calcium and phosphorus. Imbalances result in enlarged joints, inflammation of the bone growth centers (epiphysitis), sore joints, crooked legs, and occasionally, a fracture through the weakened epiphyses. Excess phosphorus diets in the pregnant mare may cause damage to the foal, which may not be corrected after birth. Such foals never mature normally. Adult horses may develop a demineralization or softening of the bones (osteomalacia). A condition known as "big head" may occur but is uncommon. Abnormal Ca:P ratios may be involved with unusual calcium deposits resulting in such conditions as ringbone, sidebones, and bone spavins. Degenerative arthritis, wobblers, and navicular disease may have this nutritional imbalance as a predisposing cause.

Muscular Problems. The whole story of "sore backs" or lumbar myositis is not clearly understood. Sore backs are evident when one puts on the saddle and the animal flinches badly and sinks down. Less obvious cases can easily be detected by applying fairly firm pressure while running the thumb and index finger down the back, over the loin area. The muscles will quiver and the horse will have a tendency to sink down. Overall skin sensitivity while using grooming brushes frequently accompanies this condition. The condition can easily be produced by giving a horse a ration of a poor-quality grass or grain hay, accompanied by a heavy grain ration of oats, barley, corn, bran, or combinations thereof. This diet has a very bad Ca:P ratio because it is quite high in phosphorus and low in calcium. Despite our basic knowledge of this problem, we too frequently see horses with sore backs while they are receiving the best balanced ration we are capable of producing. If it is a persistent problem with a given animal, it represents an unsoundness that interferes with the animal's usability.

Table VII shows typical grain mixtures that have Ca:P ration *imbalances* and Tables VIII to X show balanced grain rations for horses in various conditions of use and climate.

PELLETED FEEDS

The pelleting of feeds for all classes of livestock has become popular in recent years. The following are the pros and cons of pelleted feeds for horses.

Advantages

1. Easy storage and handling
2. Reduced dustiness

3. Easy to incorporate vitamin supplement
4. Less wastage

Disadvantages

1. Relatively more expensive
2. Predisposes horses to wood chewing
3. Too small pellets (⅝ inches or smaller) frequently cause choking
4. Cannot judge the quality of feed going into the pellets

One has to weigh these features to determine whether the pelleted feeds might work into a specific feeding program.[5]

ANTIBIOTICS IN GRAIN MIXTURES

The use of low-level antibiotics in the feed of pigs and poultry has often resulted in increased weight gains. Similar results have frequently been experienced with calves. This is probably due to the effect of the antibiotics, which prevent minor infections. Such results have not been observed when giving young colts as much as 200 mg daily of oxytetracycline hydrochloride (Henricson, B., 1960). Even more important are the findings of British workers headed by Professor M. M. Swann (The Swann Report, 1971) in England, who found that the feeding of low-level antibiotics to livestock may actually cause a public health problem by causing resistant bacteria to develop that might be pathogenic to man. These workers have demonstrated that it may be possible for nonpathogenic resistant strains to mutate to highly dangerous pathogens. Because of these findings and the lack of evidence that the feeding of antibiotics to horses has any beneficial effect, their use in feeds is not recommended and should be discouraged. The author has also experienced poor therapeutic response from the use of oxytetracycline in horses with severe respiratory infections that have been fed low levels of this antibiotic in their grain.

ENERGY AND GRAIN REQUIREMENTS FOR WORK

As an automobile needs gasoline to operate, the horse needs fuel to function. The type of work required of the horse has an overall effect on its longevity. The harder the work it performs, the greater are its feed requirements. Research has established the amount of energy that is used up during various kinds of horse activities. We express these energy requirements in terms

---

[5]The alfalfa hay wafers seem very neat and have all the advantages stated for pelleted feeds, though some are very difficult to break open. They often are a problem for older horses with dental problems. The author feels the disadvantages outweigh the advantages.

of megacalories per hour per 1000 pounds (Mcal/hr./1000 lb.). When we convert this to approximate pounds of grain needed per hour of activity, it is easier to discuss and understand. Table XIII indicates the approximate amount of balanced grain mixture needed as a supplement to a good hay ration to meet the energy requirements for these activities.

Although the figures shown in Table XIII represent a relationship between energy used and the amount of grain needed for work per hour, the final total amount of grain needed for a workout or training period cannot be figured on the basis of the sum total for the amount of time spent at each gait. Some horses are in better condition than others and thus use their energy more efficiently. The final amount of grain needed for a workout period should be based on an arbitrary estimated classification of the total work period as being light, medium, heavy, or strenuous. Table XIV is a chart that gives general recommendations. These are guidelines to help owners avoid underfeeding working animals. Skinny, drawnout, gaunt horses should not be mistaken as "fit" animals.

COMMON WORK SCHEDULES AND GRAIN REQUIREMENTS

Horse Show Equitation—Hack Work

Rail work includes working on each gait to improve it for showing; also, work on transitions from one gait to another.

Individual work includes figure eights, working on simple changes of lead, flying changes, pick up leads on straight line down center of ring, and so forth.

Light workout—30 minutes
Rail work—15 minutes
    5 minutes—walk
    5 minutes—trot
    5 minutes—canter
Individual work—15 minutes
    5 minutes—walk
    5 minutes—trot
    5 minutes—canter
Total grain—30 minutes at light work: 1 lb.

Medium workout—60 minutes
Rail work—30 minutes
    10 minutes—walk
    10 minutes—trot
    10 minutes—canter

Individual work—30 minutes
   10 minutes—walk
   10 minutes—trot
   10 minutes—canter
Total grain for 60 minutes of medium work: 3 lb.

Jumping

The warmup should include trotting and cantering.
Gymnastics work includes halts, shoulder-in, backup, trot cavalletti work, and canter cavalletti work; maximum height for just gymnastics is 3 feet 6 inches.

Light workout—30 minutes
15 minutes warmup
   10 minutes—trot
   5 minutes—canter
15 minutes gymnastics
   5 minutes—walk
   5 minutes—trot
   5 minutes—canter
Total grain: 1 lb.

Medium workout—45 minutes
15 minutes warmup
   10 minutes—trot
   5 minutes—canter
30 minutes gymnastics
   5 minutes—walk
   15 minutes—trot
   10 minutes—canter
Total grain: 2 lb.

Heavy workout—60 minutes
15 minutes warmup
   10 minutes—trot
   5 minutes—canter
45 minutes—gymnastics
   10 minutes—walk
   20 minutes—trot
   15 minutes—canter
Total grain: 8 lb.

Three-Day Event Conditioning

Light workout—20 minutes
   10 minutes—trot
   5 minutes—canter

5 minutes—trot
Total grain: ½ lb.

Medium workout—30 minutes
    10 minutes—trot
    5 minutes—canter
    10 minutes—trot
    5 minutes—canter
Total grain: 2 lb.

Heavy workout—60 minutes
    10 minutes—trot
    10 minutes—canter
    5 minutes—walk
    10 minutes—trot
    10 minutes—canter
    5 minutes—walk
    10 minutes—trot
Total grain: 8 lb.

Dressage

The warmup should include trotting and cantering.
Work consists of extended walk, shoulder-in, halts, back, circles, half pirouettes, and so forth.

Below Third Level

Light workout—30 minutes
10 minutes warmup
    5 minutes—trot
    5 minutes—canter
20 minutes dressage
    5 minutes—walk
    10 minutes—trot
    5 minutes—canter
Total grain: 1 lb.

Medium workout—45 minutes
15 minutes warmup
    10 minutes—trot
    5 minutes—canter
30 minutes dressage
    5 minutes—walk
    15 minutes—trot
    10 minutes—canter
Total grain: 2 lb.

Heavy workout—60 minutes
15 minutes warmup:
   10 minutes—trot
    5 minutes—canter
45 minutes dressage:
   10 minutes—walk
   20 minutes—trot
   15 minutes—canter
Total grain: 8 lb.

Third Level and Above

Light workout—20 minutes
5 minutes warmup:
   3 minutes—trot
   2 minutes—canter
15 minutes dressage:
   5 minutes—walk
   5 minutes—trot
   5 minutes—canter
Total grain: 1 lb.

Medium workout—30 minutes
10 minutes warmup
   5 minutes—trot
   5 minutes—canter
20 minutes dressage
   5 minutes—walk
  10 minutes—trot
   5 minutes—canter
Total grain: 2 lb.

Heavy workout—45 minutes
15 minutes warmup
  10 minutes—trot
   5 minutes—canter
30 minutes dressage
   5 minutes—walk
  15 minutes—trot
  10 minutes—canter
Total grain: 6 lb.

ENDURANCE RIDES

Conditioning

There is no one, single method of proper conditioning, but a period of at least 8 to 12 weeks should be taken for the preparation for an endurance ride. All such animals should be at least 5 years old. The walk is a very good conditioning gait and should constitute the major part of the conditioning program. Horses are often "legged up" by working them late in the program in sand at the beach. Many horses are also "swum" to help muscles get in condition. Swimming horses is a popular conditioning procedure.

A general training formula, such as the following, is commonly used but it should be noted that variations in the training program will help keep it more interesting to horse and rider.

Walk—15 minutes
Trot—10 minutes
Canter—5 minutes

The length of the conditioning period is gradually increased. Table XV is a typical schedule.

It is always wise to have the horse undergo a general physical examination by a veterinarian prior to any serious training program. Proper parasite control, dental care, and nutrition are critically important for endurance animals.

Water Balance

The most important requirement for prolonged physical exertion is maintaining proper water balance in the body. Although the horse can lose all its body fat and half its body protein, the loss of only 12 to 15% of its total body water can be fatal. To prevent this during prolonged physical activity, the horse should be encouraged to drink frequently all the water it wants. After strenuous activity, the horse may be allowed to eat hay, but should be "cooled out" (allowed to rest for 60 to 90 minutes) before it is allowed to drink an unlimited amount of cold water at will. Allowing a hot horse to drink an unlimited amount of cold water can result in founder (laminitis) and possibly colic. If the watering places on an endurance ride are more than 2 hours apart, especially if the weather is hot, it is advisable to carry 1 to 2 gallons of water with you and a collapsible pail to allow for in-between watering.

Electrolytes

During strenuous physical activity, body salts or electrolytes are lost in sweat and urine. These include four important elements: sodium, potassium, chloride, and calcium. The loss of these first three electrolytes causes muscle weakness and fatigue and a decreased interest in drinking. During an endurance ride, there is a routine loss of electrolytes, and dehydration does occur.

To prevent the harmful effects of this, electrolytes should be given and water should be offered frequently.

The amount of electrolytes lost varies under different conditions and between individual horses under similar circumstances. Because prolonged strenuous exertion does result in electrolyte loss and the giving of electrolytes causes no harm as long as water is available, it is advisable to give electrolytes to all horses that participate in endurance rides.

An inexpensive electrolyte mixture is as follows: Three tablespoons "Lite" salt and one tablespoon limestone in one gallon of water. Lite salt is a low-sodium salt that can be purchased at the grocery store and limestone is calcium carbonate. It can be purchased at most feed stores. Two ounces of this mixture can be added to a couple of ounces of water, molasses, or applesauce and squirted into the back of the horse's mouth, or it may be added to a little grain. Do not put it into the drinking water because this may reduce water consumption. This should be given before the ride, at each watering, and after the ride. Although the giving of electrolytes is advisable, the adequate intake of water is much more important.

Thumps

Another condition that may result from electrolyte loss is so-called "thumps." It results from decreased plasma calcium and/or potassium. This causes a synchronized spasm of the diaphragm (SDF—Synchronized Diaphragmatic Flutter). The horse suddenly has rhythmic movements of the flanks and sometimes a hind leg with each beat of the heart. It is believed that the phrenic nerve that goes to the diaphragm is irritated as it passes over the heart, resulting in these spasms. This condition often accompanies other symptoms of exhaustion, and veterinary care is indicated.

Training of Yearlings

In the racing world, distance is more commonly used as a unit of work than time. As a rule, it takes about three months of basic fundamental training ("breaking") before a yearling is ready for the first workouts at the track. Much walking is commonly used in the early training and the animal usually walks 2 to 3 miles daily. Slow "breezes" or galloping will be started over ⅛ of a mile (1 furlong). As the trainer decides the young horses are progressing, the breezes will be extended over a longer distance at 3- or 4-day intervals. A 1-mile gallop is scheduled daily.

Early workouts of more than ⅛ of a mile will last about 14 or 15 seconds. Animals should always be started slowly. This pace will then be extended over 4 furlongs and then gradually into the mile at 3- to 4-day intervals. The young horses should be constantly and closely examined for any evidence of lameness or injury. Then come workouts of 2 furlongs at 25 or 26 seconds with slower third and fourth furlongs. Gradually, faster times are sought over these same distances.

Training 2-Year-Olds

Young 2-year-olds are "breezed" over a half-mile in 50 seconds to give the trainer a chance to evaluate the animal. Early races should be from 3 to 5½ furlongs long. By late fall, a colt is often raced over a distance of $1^1/_{16}$ miles.

Prior to a race, the animal is usually only worked in open breeze about 7 to 10 days before the race. It is then let out at a fast breeze over 3 furlongs 1 or 2 days before the race. Older horses are allowed a sharp breeze at 3 to 4 furlongs a day or two before the race to keep fit. Amounts of grain needed for these activities can be estimated from the work-grain chart, basing the estimate on the intensity of the work at different stages of training.

RECOMMENDED FEEDING PROGRAMS

Nursing Foal to Weaning—5 or 6 Months

In the first 6 months of life, the foal grows to 77% of its mature height and 44% of its mature weight. By the time it is 1 year old, it should have reached 90% of its mature height and 60% of its mature weight. It can be seen how important this period is to a growing foal. At no other time will it have such a growth potential, and studies indicate that if it is significantly held back at this time, it will never develop to its full potential (Figs. 58, 59, and 60).

This growth potential cannot be met by even a very heavy milk-producing mare. Milk is low in iron and in certain amino acids that are needed for growth. By the time the foal is only 3 weeks old, a *creep feed* (an area where the foal can eat at will away from the mare) should be made available. A well-balanced, high-protein (18 to 20% crude protein) grain mixture should be fed. Grain feeds under 16% crude protein have been shown to limit maximum growth. As a general rule, a foal should consume 1 pound of grain per month of life (e.g., at 2 months of age, it should be eating 2 pounds of grain). This grain ration should continue to increase until the foal is receiving 6 to 8 pounds of grain per day. It is leveled off at this amount and feeding is continued at this level until the age of 2 years. Adjustments can be made depending on how well the colt appears to be developing. If a colt is in a good state of health and not anemic or heavily parasitized, it should have no trouble consuming this amount of grain. After

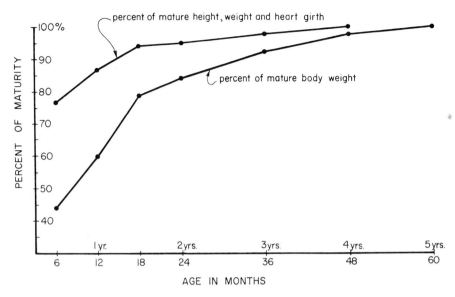

FIG. 58. Equine growth rate.

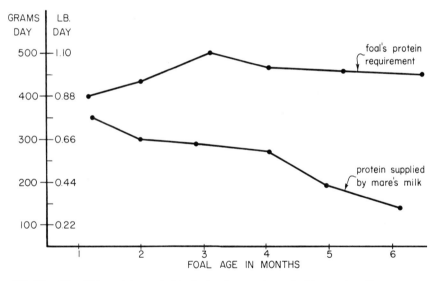

FIG. 59. Digestible protein needed by foal and amount supplied in mare's milk.

the age of 2 years, a 12 to 14% crude protein grain mixture may be used satisfactorily.

The foal should be given as much alfalfa hay and a mixture of alfalfa meal and molasses as it wants in the creep-feed area, along with a vitamin supplement. A 4-month-old foal should be getting at least 40,000 international units (i.u.) of vitamin A daily. The

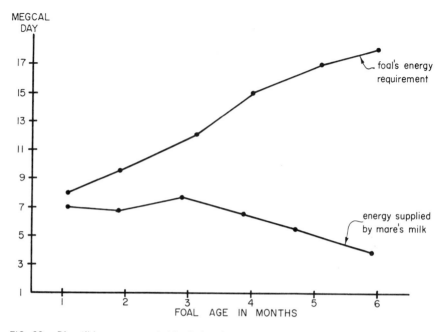

FIG. 60.   Digestible energy needed by foal and amount supplied in mare's milk.

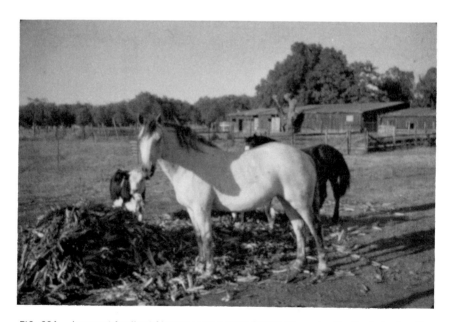

FIG. 60A.   Incorrect feeding of horses causes acute indigestion and colic, if not also founder.

mixture of alfalfa meal and molasses has some unidentified ingredients that greatly help growth and the putting on of weight.
Three to five pounds per day is a common amount consumed by
a 4-month-old foal.

In general, because horses are simple-stomached animals, it is
best to divide the feedings into two or three times daily; a horse
makes better use of its feed this way. Salt, fresh clean water, and
trace minerals—when needed—should always be available free
choice. Trace-mineral salt blocks are usually satisfactory for this
need.

A creep-feed area for a single foal should be at least 10 × 10
feet and much larger if several foals are to use the area. A simple
creep can be made by placing a low board over the entrance to a
stall. A corner of a corral can be used by constructing two sections
of fence that come out and nearly meet, leaving approximately
an 18-in. "doorway" into the feed area. This narrow entrance
makes it impossible for the mare to come in and eat the foal's
feed. The feed manger in the creep feed should be placed in the
corner that does not allow or encourage the mare to attempt to
reach it over or under the fence. If the feed seems at all reachable,
many mares will get low on their knees or push hard over the
fence in an effort to reach the feed.

The Orphan Foal

The mare's first milk, *colostrum*, is high in antibodies and is very
beneficial in giving the foal resistance against common bacterial
infection. If this is available, it should be given to the foal, but
after it is over 24 hours old, this milk, like other milk, has only
nutritional value.

A common milk formula for the orphan foal is: 20 ounces of
regular cow's milk, 12 ounces of water (lime water is desirable
because it makes cow's milk more easily digested for very young
foals), and 4 tablespoons of corn syrup. This formula should be
warmed to body temperature.

Borden's Foal-Lac is an excellent milk substitute. Straight goat's
milk may also be used satisfactorily. An adopted nurse mare
would make the problem of raising an orphan foal much easier.

Start feeding the foal within 6 to 8 hours using a lamb's nipple
on a coke bottle or similar container. Care should be taken not to
make the hole in the nipple too large, which would allow the milk
to flow faster than the foal would be able to drink. Feed the foal
only while it is standing or lying up on its chest. Never feed it
while it is lying on its side where it would be difficult for it to
swallow properly (this avoids the possibility of the milk entering
the lungs). Feed at hourly intervals for the first three days (not

feeding from 11 PM to 6 AM is not harmful). Most important during this night period is to keep the foal warm in a stall or suitable enclosure with a heat lamp or other means of warmth. Chilling, especially from cold drafts, is very stressful for any newborn animal.

After the first 3-day period, the feedings can be at 2-hour intervals during the day and gradually limited to 4 times daily by the time the foal is 1-month-old. The average foal will need about 1 pint of milk per 10 pounds of body weight per day (e.g., an 80-pound foal should receive 8 pints daily). Some foals consume considerably more than this. The foal should be taught to drink from a pail as soon as possible. After three weeks, the corn syrup can be discontinued from the milk formula.

If diarrhea occurs, reduce the milk consumption and use nonfat milk in the formula. The administration of 2 ounces of Koalin-pectate 3 times daily for 1 or 2 days may be needed. Acute watery diarrhea accompanied by a loss of appetite should receive veterinary attention as soon as possible.

By the age of 8 weeks, the liquid milk can be stopped and an equivalent amount of powdered milk can be added to the grain. Feed good alfalfa hay free choice along with the mixture of alfalfa meal and molasses. A balanced grain of 18 to 20% crude protein should be started as early as possible and should be given at the rate of 1 pound per 1 month of life as is done for other foals. Lysine, an essential amino acid found in milk, is necessary for maximum growth; powdered milk in the grain may therefore prove very worthwhile.

As with all foals, a good worming program should be started by the age of 8 weeks and continued as outlined in the discussion of a parasite control program.

Pregnant Mares

Recent studies indicate that a well-balanced ration is very important in early pregnancy, but the total quantity of feed doesn't rise significantly above that needed by an idle mature horse. During the last quarter of pregnancy, the foal attains 75% of its growth. An adequate source of vitamins (especially vitamin A—35,000 to 50,000 i.u./day) is necessary for proper growth of the bones and tendons of the foal. Excess phosphorus rations can cause harmful bone effects that may result in the foal's never reaching proper maturity. Since the vitamin A content of a given feed is unreliable because it oxidizes readily in storage, it is always wise to give a vitamin supplement in the grain.

A ration of 15 pounds of good-quality hay (at least half alfalfa is recommended) with 2 to 4 pounds of 12 to 14% crude protein is normally adequate to meet the pregnant mare's nutritional needs.

It should be part of basic good husbandry to have the pregnant mare on a conscientious worming program, especially in the period of 4 to 6 weeks before foaling. All foals eat the manure of the mare, and by having her as free of parasites as possible, the foal has a better chance at early development and may prevent early cases of diarrhea in the foal.

It is also good to have the mare's teeth floated and have her in as good condition as possible at foaling time to help assure her chances of producing a healthy foal and an adequate milk supply. Though it is not advisable to have a mare excessively fat at foaling time, rarely does this cause a problem.

Mature Idle Horses

No grain is actually required for most horses that are used less than an hour per day, but 1 or 2 pounds of grain a day gives them something to look forward to. Feed about 15 pounds (two 4-inch flakes) of good-quality hay per day. Alfalfa hay is an excellent hay for horses and is commonly fed as the only source of hay. The feeding of alfalfa frequently corrects the imbalance of many grain rations. One feeding of alfalfa and one of oat or other good-quality hay adds variety to the horse's diet. Though many areas have good pasture that can sustain horses very well, it should be realized that when pastures become mature and very dry, their nutritional value (especially vitamins and protein content) is greatly reduced. At this time, the horse's diet should be supplemented with good-quality feed. Even though many animals appear fat while feeding on a mature dry-grass pasture, this is not an indication that the animal is well nourished. Such pastures only have carbohydrate value. Many horses drop off in condition rapidly when they are expected to overwinter on such pastures. These animals are on a starvation diet.

Horses at Light to Strenuous Work

These horses should receive from 4 to 12 pounds of grain daily plus 15 pounds of hay. Half alfalfa and half oat or similar hay is sufficient. Some horses are harder keepers than others and thus should be fed accordingly. See Tables XIII and XIV to estimate needs for various amounts of work. Stallions are fed like other working horses. Total amounts vary according to the frequency of their use.

Nursing Mares

Many good nursing mares will produce 40 pounds (5 gallons) of milk per day—the same as a good dairy cow. Mare owners are too frequently unaware of the high nutritional requirements that are necessary to maintain this high rate of production. Because of this, many nursing mares are badly underfed and severely drop off in weight and condition. The hay ration should be one flake (4 to 5 inches thick) of alfalfa hay twice daily. A ration of one-half oat hay will give the diet variety and is satisfactory. Since there is a gradual increase in milk production coinciding with the growth of the foal, the grain ration is increased accordingly. The following is a suitable schedule:

Foaling through first 4 weeks post-foaling 2–4 lbs. grain daily
2 months post-foaling . . . . 4–6 lb. grain daily
3 months post-foaling . . . . 6–8 lb. grain daily
4 months post-foaling . . . . 8–10 lb. grain daily
5 months post-foaling to weaning. . . . . . . 10–12 lb. grain daily

After weaning, the mare is fed according to her needs at that time. This depends on her activities and general condition.

Underweight Horses

There is a common general misconception that many horses are just "hard keepers" and can never be fattened. This is very rarely the case except for certain diseased horses. Almost *any* horse, despite his age, can be kept in good flesh. Again, don't be fooled by a horse that has a "big belly." Horses that are underweight characteristically have little or no flesh over their withers, over their ribs, or over the croup (pelvis). Such animals usually have a dry, long haircoat that is greasy at its base. This long haircoat may cover the ribs so that it is difficult to see how skinny the horse really is. Such an animal definitely needs help and a specific fattening diet is necessary for it to regain its general condition in any reasonably short period of time. First, it is important that the animal be treated for both internal and external parasites. The horse should also have its teeth floated.

A common fattening diet is:

1. One flake (4 inches thick, approximately 8 pounds) of alfalfa hay twice daily. (One feeding of good-quality oat hay is acceptable.)
2. Three to four 2-pound coffee cans (they only hold a little over a pound of grain) of a well-balanced grain mixture.
3. One bucket (13 quarts) of alfalfa meal and molasses once or twice daily.

4. A good vitamin supplement once daily.

On this diet, almost any horse will put on flesh and regain a good general condition in 6 to 8 weeks. At that time, this diet can be markedly reduced to meet the horse's new maintenance and work requirements. It should be emphasized that to prevent digestive upsets, a change in the feeding program should be done over a 4- to 7-day period.

An alternate fattening diet that is very satisfactory and safe is the same hay ration as mentioned in the previous diet, but with about one-third to one-half the grain suggested and free choice alfalfa meal and molasses (i.e., place a large drum filled with alfalfa meal and molasses in with the horse, thus allowing it to eat as much as it wants). Because this is only hay ground up with molasses, it is safe to feed it in this manner.[6] Underweight horses usually eat about 100 pounds in the first 3 days and then start leveling off the amount they eat. Needless to say, horses on either of these special diets need to be fed by themselves. One common reason for underweight horses, aside from not being fed enough, is more aggressive horses in a pasture preventing them from getting their daily ration.

Horses on this diet "bloom" very quickly and are often back in good flesh in only 3 weeks. Many old horses with bad teeth are maintained on this ration at all times. It should be noted that this alternate fattening diet is best utilized for those horses that become very high and nervous on heavy grain rations.

It should again be noted that only good-quality feed should be fed to horses; defective feeds can cause acute digestive upsets and serious colic (Fig. 60A).

Overweight Horses

Overweight horses are often the most difficult problem to handle. Some horses, especially ponies, Arabians, and Morgans, are very easy keepers and it often seems that one almost has to starve them to get them down to a "normal" weight. Many horses are truly hypothyroid animals, and it is advisable to have a veterinarian examine an animal for this condition if it is suspected. Clinically, hypothyroid animals develop very large firm crests (of the neck) and have fat deposits over their shoulders and back. These animals have a tendency to founder easily—especially on plush spring grass—and the mares are difficult to get into foal. "Grass founder" seems to occur only in hypothyroid animals.

A ration of good-quality oat, timothy, or similar hay that is

---

[6]Of course, grain can never be given free choice to horses.

bulky, but lower in TDN, is indicated. Give 10 to 15 pounds per day, depending on the results. One pound of grain may be given because that quantity is never more than a treat and provides a means of getting needed vitamins into the diet. Veterinarians are able to give specific recommendations.

The Aged Horse

The aged horse often does not require a special type of feeding, unless it is having difficulty maintaining its weight. This is usually the result of dental problems. After a horse is 20 years old, it is especially important that it have frequent dental examinations and care. Many such animals need their teeth filed at 6-month intervals, which may also be the case for much younger horses. When teeth are lost or the animal develops very irregular chewing surfaces on its teeth, chewing becomes very difficult. As a result, much of the nutritional value of the feed is lost because it depends on thorough chewing for efficient digestion of nutrients.

Two common indications that a horse's teeth are bad is excessive feed dropping out of the mouth while the horse is eating and the history of a horse getting very fat on green pastures, but "falling off" in flesh badly when put on dry feed. Slowness of eating is another sign, with or without excessive salivation.

To compensate for these problems, we feed a diet consisting mostly of ground hays (15 to 18 pounds daily) along with whatever amount of well-balanced grain is necessary to maintain their weight (usually 8 to 10 pounds daily). Alfalfa meal and molasses is suitable roughage and can constitute most of the diet of the aged horse.

If the animal is down in weight, it is best to follow the general suggestions for an underweight horse, but give a larger amount of the hay portion as alfalfa meal and molasses (10 to 15 pounds daily). With age in horses, there is frequently a less resilient intestinal tract. This, coupled with poor teeth, predisposes the animal to constipation or impactions. A bran mash given once or twice a week is beneficial for such animals.

Without a doubt, one of the most inhumane acts people commonly do to old horses is to "turn them out to pasture." This usually means they are turned out on 40 acres of dirt with hardly any teeth left in their heads and are expected to make it on their own; such animals are just turned out to die and usually do so of starvation. Aged horses, like aged people, usually need extra attention; unless such horses are being retired to a permanent green, lush pasture, such acts of "good will" should be re-evaluated.

WINTER FEEDING AND CARE OF HORSES

The proper feeding and maintenance of horses in the winter requires a thorough understanding of special conditions that occur during that time of the year. These conditions markedly affect the overall well-being of horses and thus the necessary husbandry procedure should be instituted in order to meet their special needs and to keep them in a good state of health. These factors include:

1. During *cold weather,* a horse's maintenance requirements are increased in order to maintain normal body heat.
2. *External parasites* (ticks and lice) reach their peak annual population level and thus inflict severe stress on parasitized animals, causing marked blood loss, weakness, and lowered resistance.
3. *Winter pastures* of old dry grass stubble and early grass have little if any nutritional value. As pasture grasses mature and dry up, they lose almost all protein and vitamin value. They only represent a source of carbohydrates. Unlike cattle, which have an active bacterial "vat" (the rumen) in which poor-quality feed can be made into good-quality feed, horses must receive a continual supply of good feed in order to meet their normal maintenance requirements. Early winter grasses are mostly water and must mature more to develop "strength." In northern California, pastures are markedly deficient in basic nutrients that meet the needs of horses from about the middle of August to the middle of February. If horses are turned out on such pastures, they are literally on a starvation diet. Large amounts of the dry stubble allow many horses to maintain their body weight, but such animals are in a malnutritious state. Horses should be supplemented (fed as if in a corral) during the winter and such excuses as "they are range animals" to rationalize their not being fed are not acceptable. Horse owners who "turn them out for the winter" are truly abandoning their responsibilities to properly care for their animals and should be subject to laws prohibiting the inhumane treatment of animals. Though it is true that many animals in the wild must survive under these conditions, this does not justify man's inflicting this situation on his domestic animals.
4. *Old horses,* especially with bad teeth, need to have special diets of easily digested feed all year long. Such animals are those especially noted to "fall off" in flesh when forced out on winter pastures with these as their only source of nutrition.
5. *Pregnant mares* need to be properly fed with a balanced ration

and vitamin supplement in order to ensure the delivery of a healthy, well-developed foal.

6. *Horses' feet* continue to grow throughout the winter as they do throughout the rest of the year and they still need routine care (trimmed at least every 8 weeks, and some as often as every 6 weeks). Even if a horse's shoes are pulled and left off for the winter, routine trimming of the feet is still necessary to prevent hooves from splitting, deep thrush, and strained tendons. Horses that are forced to stand in deep mud for long periods of time (often weeks) are very susceptible to thrush, a thin and scurfy condition of the heels ("dish pan hands"), and to mud fever, which is an infectious dermatitis of the skin of the lower legs. These conditions should be prevented by providing all horses with some area that is well drained or out of the mud where they can stand and allow their feet to dry out.

   If a horse must be kept in a pasture or corral area with no shelter, then a large area (allowing at least an area of 15 × 15 feet for each horse) or platform should be constructed for this purpose. Such a platform can be made by framing the selected area with outer 4 × 4 inch posts and inner bracing with 4 × 4 posts and filling it in with river rock or road base. Allow plenty of space between feeding areas for the horses to prevent fighting and injuries.

7. A *shelter* of some kind is strongly recommended for horses, especially in the winter. Though a closed-in stable or barn is desirable, even a three-sided shelter can offer comfort from the wind and weather. Despite the fact that many horses can survive out in the elements, this does not negate the value of providing a shelter. Such a facility should have a minimum space of 12 × 12 feet and preferably 14 × 14 feet. A barn or stable can be a necessity for horses during times of illness or recovery from an injury. Heat lamps or blankets can offer much comfort to horses during the winter. Always clean the stable daily and keep it well bedded.

8. *Shivering* (see page 255).

9. Horses are *more susceptible* to respiratory infections and the effects of external and internal parasites. Giving horses proper care during these months is imperative in maintaining good health.

   As can be seen from the discussion of the special conditions that occur during the winter, horses should have very close attention given to them and their needs so that they can be kept and enjoyed in good health all year long.

GENERAL FEEDING NOTES

1. Horses have simple stomachs and make better use of frequent feedings. The daily ration should be divided into at least two feedings.
2. Horses depend partly on the bacteria in the digestive tract to assist digestion. These bacteria have to adjust to changes in feed. Sudden changes in a ration may cause indigestion and colic. Always introduce changes in the diet gradually over a 4- to 7-day period.
3. Be able to recognize a horse in poor flesh and condition by the loss of muscling along the sides of the withers and over the croup. Such horses usually have prominent ribs, but a long, shaggy coat may make the ribs less evident. Don't mistake a horse with a "hay belly" for a fat horse.
4. A diet of a large amount of a poor quality hay can be heavy in the digestive tract and press against the diaphragm. This reduces the horse's breathing efficiency and can cause labored breathing and quick tiring.
5. The common causes of a "pot belly" or "sprung ribs" are (a) a large intake of poor-quality hays or pasture; (b) insufficient protein in ration; (c) parasitism; and (d) a combination of these factors.
6. A lack of bulk or too much grain can result in colic from indigestion and impactions and may cause wood chewing.
7. Overfeeding of grain predisposes to laminitis. Free choice hay or alfalfa meal and molasses causes no problems.
8. Alfalfa hay is not hard on the kidneys, though it does stimulate more urination. It is not too "hot" a feed nor will it "burn a horse out." It does not specifically cause excess sweating unless the horse has become overly fat from eating too much and is out of condition. If it is cut too early, it may cause diarrhea. Some individual horses are allergic to alfalfa hay and should be fed other good roughage.
9. Defective feeds (moldy, dusty, musty, full of foxtails or bearded barley, weedy) should not be fed to the horse because they may cause severe colic or mouth wounds. If a handful of hay cannot be crushed without its causing pain or injury to the hand, it is too coarse and abrasive to use. When considering the possibility of a feed being defective, it is wise to follow the rule, "If in doubt, throw it out."
10. Storing feeds with too much moisture can cause premature oxidation of the ingredients, thus lowering its nutritional value, and molding usually results. Hays may go through a "sweat" and such bales can generate much heat and occa-

sionally cause a fire. If such hot bales are immediately opened and sprinkled with coarse salt, the hay may be saved. Bales having gone through such a sweat are usually very heavy, have no bounce when dropped, are faded brown, and are very dusty and musty from mold spores. The general quality of hay is judged by its color, fineness of stem, leafiness or amount of grain it contains, amount of foreign material, and freedom from dust.

FEEDING MAXIMS

1. Feed horses according to their requirements, which depend on their growth, production, or work performance. Reduce rations when work is reduced.
2. Never fail to observe the condition of the animal. If the horse is too thin, correct the causes and feed more. If the animal is too fat, reduce its feed according to a veterinarian's advice.
3. Feed at least twice daily. This increases horses' feed utilization.
4. Maintain regular feeding times.
5. Provide unlimited good, clean water at all times, unless the animal is overheated.
6. Provide sanitary watering and feeding conditions.
7. Water, hay, and grain may be fed at any time in relation to each other. Watering before or after feeding does not interfere with the digestion of either the grain or the hay.
8. Avoid sudden changes in the feeding program. Adjust changes in the diet over a 4- to 7-day period.
9. Allow an hour or more after feeding before hard work.
10. Do not feed grain to tired or hot horses or allow unlimited water. Hay, on the other hand, will not harm them.
11. Do not allow other horses to prevent an individual from getting its full ration.
12. *Never* give a horse moldy, spoiled, or questionable feed.

TABLE I. Comparing Concentrates (under 12% crude fiber)

Feed	Crude protein, %	Cost/sack	Cost/100 lb	Cost/lb crude protein
Commercial mix #1	14	$ 9.25/50 lb	$18.50	$1.32
Commercial mix #2	12	8.75/50 lb	17.50	1.45
Oats, rolled	8.7	11.00/75 lb	14.66	1.68

Mix #1	Costs $18.50/100 lb bag, which contains 14% or 14 lb of crude protein. Thus, $18.50 ÷ 14 = $1.32/lb crude protein.
Mix #2	Costs $17.50/100 lb, which contains 12% or 12 lb crude protein. Thus, $17.50 ÷ 12 = $1.45/lb crude protein.
Oats, rolled	Cost $14.66/100 lb, which contains 8.7% or 8.7 lb crude protein. Thus, $14.66 ÷ 8.7 = $1.68/lb crude protein.
Results:	Mix #1 is the best buy based on crude protein, even though it costs the most per 100 lb — the difference between cost and value.
Note:	Although the cost of protein is important, more important is that the mix has a *balanced calcium-phosphorus ratio*. If it does not, it can cause muscle and bone problems. Also, if the mix contains a vitamin-mineral supplement, this substantially increases its value.

TABLE II. Comparing Roughages (over 25% crude fiber)

Feed	Crude protein, %	Cost/unit	Cost/100 lb	Cost/lb crude protein
Commercial mix: Hay and grain pelleted together	12	$ 14.50/100 lb	$14.50	$1.21
Alfalfa hay	17.5	159.00/ton	7.95	45¢
Alfalfa hay cubed	17.5	7.95/70 lb	11.36	65¢
Oat hay	7.5	120.00/ton	6.00	80¢
Alfalfa meal and molasses	15.0	6.95/5 lb	13.90	93¢

Commercial mix	Costs $14.50/100 lb for 12 lb (12%) crude protein. $14.50 ÷ 12 = 1.21/lb crude protein.
Alfalfa hay	Costs $7.95/100 lb for 17.5 lb (17.5%) crude protein. $7.95 ÷ 17.5 = 45¢/lb crude protein.
Alfalfa hay cubed	Costs $11.36 for 17.5 lb (17.5%) crude protein. $11.36 ÷ 17.5 = 65¢/lb crude protein.
Oat hay	Costs $6.00/100 lb for 7.5 lb (7.5%) crude protein. $6.00 ÷ 7.5 = 80¢/lb crude protein.
Alfalfa meal and molasses	Cost $13.90 for 15 lb (15%) crude protein. $13.90 ÷ 15 = 93¢/lb crude protein.
Result:	Based on crude protein, alfalfa hay is by far the best buy.
Note:	Oat hay cost of crude protein is almost twice that of alfalfa hay, although the cost per ton is less.

TABLE III. Comparing Vitamin A Content of Commercial Vitamin Mixtures

	Vitamin A u/lb	Cost/u	Cost/lb	Cost/100,000 u
Mix #1	22,000	$43.95/22 lb	$2.00	$9.09
Mix #2	40,000	35.95/50 lb	.72	1.80
Mix #3	110,000	25.85/25 lb	1.03	.94
Mix #4	600,000	27.95/25 lb	1.12	.19

Mix #1 costs $2.00 for   22,000 u. Thus: 100,000 u cost $2.00 ÷ .22 = $9.09.
Mix #2 costs   .72 for 40,000 u. Thus: 100,000 u cost   .72 ÷ .4 = 1.80.
Mix #3 costs 1.03 for 110,000 u. Thus: 100,000 u cost 1.03 ÷ 1.1 =   .94.
Mix #4 costs 1.12 for 600,000 u. Thus: 100,000 u cost 1.12 ÷ 6   =   .19.

Result: As can be seen, there is a wide range of cost. To merit such a cost gap, a product should have ample clinical evidence of its value over other mixes available, not just a good advertising campaign.

TABLE IV. Feed Values of Common Feeds[a]

Concentrates:	TDN, %	Dig. Prot., %	DM, %	Ca, %	P, %	Ca:P (approx.)
Oats	72.2	7.0	91.2	0.09	0.34	1:3.5
Barley	78.7	6.9	89.8	0.06	0.37	1:6
Corn	80.1	6.6	85.2	0.02	0.27	1:11
Linseed meal	77.2	30.8	91.0	0.33	0.86	1:2.5
Cottonseed meal	78.4	36.4	92.7	0.23	1.12	1:5
Soybean meal	78.6	37.5	90.9	0.30	0.67	1:2
Bran	67.2	13.7	90.1	0.14	1.29	1:9
Molasses	54.0	0	74.0	0.74	0.08	9:1
Roughages:						
Alfalfa hay	50.3	10.6	90.5	1.43	0.21	7:1
Oat hay	46.3	4.5	88.1	0.22	0.17	1:1
Timothy hay	46.9	2.9	89.0	0.27	0.16	2:1
Barley hay	51.9	4.0	90.8	0.26	0.23	1:1
Wheat hay	46.5	3.2	90.4	0.18	0.21	1:1
Sudan grass hay	48.5	4.3	89.3	.446	.036	10:1
Mature voluntary hay	49.2	2.6	90.0	0.40	0.10	4:1
Mature grass pasture	41.0	0.2	90.0	0.30	0.08	4:1
Alfalfa meal	53.6	11.8	92.7	1.32	0.19	6:1
Oat straw	44.1	0.9	89.7	0.36	0.13	3:1

[a]Information herein taken mostly from *Morrison's Feeds and Feeding,* The Morrison Publishing Co. (Ithaca, New York, 1957).

TABLE V. Horse Feed Requirements[a]

	TDN, lb.	Dig. Prot., lb.	DM, lb.	Ca	P	Ca:P
Idle	7–9	0.6–0.8	13–18	0.033	0.033	1:1
Light work	9–11	0.8–1.0	15–18	0.033	0.033	1:1
Medium work	11–13	1.0–1.2	15–18	0.033	0.033	1:1
Hard work	13–18	1.2–1.4	18–22	0.033	0.033	1:1
Last one-fourth of pregnancy	7–9	1.2–1.4	15–18	0.035	0.033	1:1
Nursing mare	14–18	1.2–1.5	18–22	0.077	0.066	1:1
500-lb. colt	6–8	0.9–1.0	10–13	0.088	0.066	1:1

[a]Ponies and work horses should be fed according to their relative body weight, using the recommendations in this table as a guideline.

Table VI. Comparison of Feed Values of Common Hays

Amount/lb.	Hay	TDN	Dig. Prot.	DM	Ca	P	Ca:P
15	Alfalfa	7.5	1.6	13.6	0.22	0.036	6:1
15	Oat	7.0	0.68	13.2	0.033	0.026	1:1
15	Timothy	7.0	0.43	13.0	0.040	0.024	2:1
15	Mature volunteer	7.5	0.39	13.5	0.060	0.015	4:1

TABLE VII. Typical Grain Mixtures with Ca:P Imbalance

Grain Mixture #1

Amount/lb.	Feed	TDN, lb.	Dig. Prot., lb.	Ca	P	Ca:P
40	Oats	28.8	2.8	0.036	0.136	1:3.5
40	Barley	31.4	2.8	0.024	0.148	1:6
20	Corn	16.4	1.3	0.004	0.054	1:11
100	Mix	76.6	6.9	0.064	0.338	1:53

Grain Mixture #2

40	Oats	28.8	2.9	0.036	0.136	1:3.5
40	Barley	31.4	2.8	0.024	0.148	1:6
20	Bran	13.5	2.7	0.028	0.258	1:9
100	Mix	73.7	8.7	0.088	0.542	1:6.2

Grain Mixture #3

35	Oats	25.1	2.5	0.032	0.119	1:3.5
35	Barley	27.2	2.5	0.021	0.130	1:6
20	Bran	13.5	2.9	0.028	0.258	1:9
10	Linseed meal	7.7	3.1	0.033	0.086	1:2.5
100	Mix	73.5	11.0	0.114	0.593	1:6

Total Ration—Imbalanced

15	Oat hay	7.0	0.68	0.033	0.026	1:1
5	Grain mix #3	3.7	0.55	0.006	0.030	1:6
20	Ration	10.7	1.23	0.039	0.056	1:1.43
15	Timothy hay	7.0	0.43	0.040	0.024	2:1
6	Grain mix #2	4.4	0.52	0.053	0.033	1:6.2
21	Ration	11.4	0.95	0.093	0.057	1:1.63

TABLE VIII. Balanced Grain Ration for Working Horses in Summer— 9.4% Crude Protein

Amount, lb.	Feed	TDN, lb.	Dig. Prot., lb.	DM, lb.	Ca	P
50	Oats	36.1	3.5	45.6	0.045	0.170
25	Barley	19.7	1.7	22.4	0.015	0.092
10	Corn	8.0	0.7	8.5	0.002	0.002
15	Alfalfa meal and molasses	8.0	1.6	13.6	0.189	0.027
100	Mix	72.8	7.5	90.1	0.251	0.316

Cruce Protein = 9.4%   Digestible Protein = 7.5%   Ca:P = 1:1.2
A suitable general all around grain mixture except for horses requiring a high protein ration.

TABLE IX. Balanced Grain Ration for Working Horses in Winter—9.5% Crude Protein

Amount, lb.	OabFeed	TDN, lb.	Dig. Prot., lb.	DM, lb.	Ca	P
45	Oats	32.5	3.2	41.0	0.041	0.153
20	Barley	15.7	1.4	18.0	0.012	0.074
20	Corn	16.2	1.4	17.0	0.004	0.054
15	Alfalfa meal and molasses	8.0	1.6	13.6	0.189	0.027
100	Mix	72.4	7.6	89.6	0.246	0.308

Crude Protein = 9.5%   Digestible Protein = 7.6%   Ca:P = 1:1.2

TABLE X. Balanced Grain Ration for Growing Foals, Nursing Mares, and Show Horses—15% Crude Protein

Amount, lb.	Feed	TDN, lb.	Dig. Prot., lb.	DM, lb.	Ca	P
40	Oats	28.9	2.8	36.5	0.036	0.136
20	Barley	15.7	1.4	18.0	0.012	0.074
10	Corn	8.1	0.7	8.5	0.002	0.027
8	Soybean meal	6.3	3.0	7.3	0.026	0.069
8	Linseed meal	6.2	2.5	7.3	0.026	0.069
14	Alfalfa meal and molasses	8.0	1.6	13.6	0.189	0.027
100	Mix	73.2	12.0	91.2	0.289	0.385

Crude Protein = 15%   Digestible Protein = 12%   Ca:P = 1:1.3
A cup/day of powdered milk in the grain ration of growing foals is advisable to provide needed lysine.

TABLE XI. Guidelines for Feeding Horses
(Daily Quantity Recommended for 1000-lb. Horse[a])

Colt 2 weeks to 5 months:	*Hay:*	alfalfa hay and alfalfa meal and molasses free choice with offerings of good oat hay.
	Grain:	2 to 5 lb. (18% crude protein)
Weaning to 2-year-old:	*Hay:*	alfalfa hay 10–15 lb. with offerings of alfalfa meal and molasses and good oat hay.
	Grain:	4 to 8 lb. (18% crude protein)
Mature idle horse: (working less than 1 hr./day)	*Hay:*	half alfalfa and half oat to givbe variety, total of 15 lb.
	Grain:	None necessary but giving 1 to 2 lb. (10 to 12% crude protein) is a treat and offers a method of giving a vitamin supplement.
Horse at light work: (1 to 3 hr./day)	*Hay:*	half alfalfa and half oat for total of 15 to 18 lb.
	Grain:	4 to 6 lb. (10–12% crude protein)
Horse at medium work: (3 to 5 hr./day)	*Hay:*	half alfalfa and half oat for a total of 15 to 18 lb.
	Grain:	6 to 9 lb. (12% crude protein)
Horse at heavy work: (5 to 8 hr./day)	*Hay:*	half alfalfa and half oat for a total of 18 to 20 lb.
	Grain:	9 to 12 lb. (12% crude protein)
Pregnant mare in last quarter:	*Hay:*	half alfalfa and half oat for a total of 15 to 18 lb.; all alfalfa ok
	Grain:	2 to 4 lb. (12 to 14% crude protein)
Nursing mare:	*Hay:*	half alfalfa and half oat for a total of 18 to 20 lb.; all alfalfa ok
	Grain:	8 to 12 lb. (12 to 14% crude protein)
Breeding stallion:	*Hay:*	half alfalfa and half oat for a total of 15 to 18 lb.
	Grain:	6 to 10 lb. (12 to 14% crude protein)

[a]1. A general vitamin supplement is recommended for all horses. Vitamin A is especially important for pregnant mares and growing foals. Vitamin E is recommended for all working and breeding animals but is still controversial; 2. Alfalfa meal and molasses is a good supplement for fattening; 3. All feeding programs should be adjusted to individual animals and their needs. If an animal is underweight, increase his feed, provide dental care, and control parasites. If a horse is overweight, feed accordingly with proper concern for minimal body requirements. Ask your veterinarian for specific recommendations for weight control programs.

TABLE XII. Suggested Daily Intakes of Vitamins A, D, and E for Horses (Cunha, 1966)

	Vitamin A	Vitamin D	Vitamin E
Foals			
to 2 months	5,000	750	10
2 to 5 months	10,000	1500	20
5 to 18 months	20,000	3000	40
18 months to maturity	40,000	6000	80
Mature horse	40,000	6000	80
Barren mare	60,000	9000	120
Breeding stallion	60,000	9000	120

TABLE XIII. Grain Needed to Meet Energy Requirements[a,b]

Classification of work	Amount grain/hr. per 1000 lb., Mcal[b]	Energy used greater than walking requirement
Very light (walking)	0.15	—
Light (slow trot, some canter)	1.5	10
Medium (fast trot, canter, some jumping)	3.25	25
Heavy (canter, galloping, jumping, cutting)	7.5	47
Strenuous (racing, polo, games)	12.25	77

[a]The suggested amounts of a *balanced grain mixture* are above any feed requirements needed for normal maintenance.
[b]1 Mcal (Megacalorie) = 1000 Kcal; 1 Kcal = 1000 cal.

TABLE XIV. Work—Grain Chart—Amount of Grain (in lb.) Needed for Various Amounts of Work*

Time, min.	Work			
	Light	Medium	Heavy	Strenuous
15	⅓	1	2	3
30	¾	1½	4	6
45	1	2	6	9
60	1½	3	7½	12

[a]The grain should be markedly reduced during days of rest.

TABLE XV. Conditioning Schedule

Week	Time	Amount of grain, lb.
1st	up to 30 minutes	2
2nd	30–60 minutes	2 to 3
3rd		
4th	60–90 minutes	3 to 5
5th		
6th	2 to 3 hours	6 to 8
7th		
8th	3 to 5 hours	8 to 10
10th		
11th	5 to 8 hours	10 to 14
12th		

6

Breeding Horses

BASIC PHYSIOLOGY

Mares are "seasonal polyestrous." This means that mares have normal "heat cycles" only through part of the year, usually from early spring to late fall. In warm climates, mares may have relatively normal cycles throughout most of the year. Every 21 to 22 days the mare develops and releases (ovulates) an ovum or egg from either of her two ovaries. The ovum passes down the horn of the uterus to the main body of the uterus. If fertilization does not occur by the sperm of the stallion meeting the ovum in the horn, the ovum dies and the mare will produce another ovum in 21 days. This is called the "estrous cycle." Outwardly the estrous cycle is characterized by two phases. One phase is the "in-heat" period, during which the mare will accept the stallion for breeding. The mare will indicate her receptiveness to the stallion by her frequent urination and "winking" of the vulva when she is near the stallion. This is normally a 5- to 6-day period. The second phase of the estrous cycle is when the mare is out of heat and not receptive to the stallion. At this time the mare usually will lay back her ears, squeal, and kick out at the stallion. This is normally a 16-day period and represents the time period between "heat periods." Most often, a mare will not show her heat period unless she is around a stallion or a gelding that will "tease" her by acting interested.

If fertilization does occur after the mare is bred by the stallion, no more heat cycles should be evident until after the foal is born.

After each ovulation, the "hole" that is left in the ovary is filled

TABLE XVI.   Breeding Notes Chart[a]

Physiology of the Mare

Onset of sexual maturity (puberty)	10 to 24 months (18 months)
Average recommended age for first breeding	2 to 3 years, depending on development
Average length of estrous cycle	19 to 23 days (21 days)
Average length of heat period	4.5 to 6.5 days (5.5 days)
Usual length of time between heat periods	13 to 18 days (15 days)
Time of ovulation	1 to 2 days before the end of the heat period
Most fertile time for breeding	2nd or 3rd day of heat or 3 days before out of heat
Advisable time to breed back after foaling	2nd heat (25 to 35 days)
Life span of the ovum after leaving the ovary	2 to 6 hours
Breeding season	February through August (depending on latitude)

Physiology of the Stallion

Onset of sexual maturity	10 to 24 months (18 months)
Average recommended age for first breeding	2 to 3 years, depending on development, young males should be used conservatively
Life span of sperm in female reproductive tract	2 to 4+ days

Stud bookings (number of mares per season)

2 year old	10 to 15 (2 to 3 per week—if at all)
3 year old	15 to 20 (spread out, with rest periods)
4 year old	20 to 30 (avoid two per day "doubles")
Mature	30 to 40 (2 or 3 "doubles" a week possible)
18 to 25	10 to 20

Some stallions have served 100 mares in a season.

([a]Chart courtesy of Dr. S. J. Roberts, Ithaca, NY)

in with a special hormone-producing tissue called the "yellow body" or corpus luteum. This tissue produces a hormone called progesterone, which prevents the development of another ovum on the ovaries and quiets the normal uterine contractions in preparation for pregnancy. If the mare is not bred or does not become pregnant, the "yellow body" tissue becomes inactive and disappears. This then allows for further production of estrogen (the major female hormone) by the ovaries to produce another ovum for the next estrous cycle. If the mare does become pregnant, the production of progesterone first by the "yellow body" and later by the placenta keeps the mare from having any more "heat cycles" until about 7 to 10 days post-foaling. This is called the "foaling heat." The average length of time a mare carries a foal (the gestation period) is 345 days. Some mares (approximately 17%) will show false heat periods while they are in foal. When this occurs it usually lasts only 24 hours and seldom will a mare actually allow a stallion to breed her when she is having a false heat period while pregnant. A forced breeding at this time may induce an abortion. Physically, these false heat periods are indistinguishable from a true estrous.

STANDING A STALLION AT STUD

To maintain a stallion for breeding is not a recommended activity for the novice horseman. This is true for the following reasons: (a) most stallions are unpredictable and are always potentially dangerous (there are many exceptions to this generalization); (b) stallions should have special holding facilities—a suitable shelter and a strong fence (an electric wire inside the fence is often desirable, an exercise area of 30 × 50 feet should be considered a bare minimum with a much larger area of a quarter acre or more being even better); (c) adequate facilities are essential for incoming mares and their care is a significant responsibility; and (d) a thorough understanding of breeding physiology, hygiene, teasing, and common problems is essential for a successful and productive effort.

It is best for all those concerned—for the horses and the people—that the standing of a stallion at stud be an activity for experienced horsemen.

Breeding Procedures

Teasing

To determine what phase of the estrous cycle a mare is in, she is "teased" by allowing a stallion to be next to her. At this time she will indicate her receptiveness or rejection. Because of the need to breed a mare at the proper time in her heat cycle, the success of a breeding program can depend on a carefully carried out teasing program.

1. Maiden mares and "open" mares (those not in foal) should be teased at least 30 days prior to the breeding season; each mare's individual cycle should be recorded. These mares should be teased at least every other day until signs of heat are detected. At this time, daily teasing should be done and continued for 2 to 3 days past the time of her going out. Again, every other day teasing is done until her next heat period when she is to be bred. These teasing records can be a great help to determine the proper time for breeding or to help recognize problems when they occur.
2. Mares that have been bred are "teased back" in order to note whether the mare shows any sign of coming back in heat. These mares are often teased every 2 or 3 days following

their breeding heat cycles but are carefully teased daily over a 7-day period beginning with the sixteenth day after the mare goes out of heat. If the mare did not conceive she should be showing in heat by the eighteenth day after going out of her heat cycle (see Chart II).

3. Following foaling, mares should be teased daily, beginning on the fourth day, if ninth-day breeding is to be considered. Mares should never be bred before 9 days, and not at all in this heat period unless the mare is normal in every respect—no internal bruising, no discharge, and "clean" on bacterial culture as determined by a veterinarian. It is best to wait for the next cycle to breed back. The mare should be teased every other day from the twentieth day, and then daily from the twenty-fifth day on through the thirty-fifth day. Most mares will be showing in by the thirtieth day.

Breeding Pattern

If a mare is normal and healthy and her heat cycle has been well established by a conscientious teasing program, breeding her on the third day before she is due to go out of heat is most likely to result in conception. This is usually the third day of heat. Studies have indicated that breeding a mare 2 or more times during the heat period only increases the conception rate 3% and does increase the opportunity for infection.

Many times it is not possible to have a mare's cycle pre-established, so it is common practice to breed her on the second and fourth days of her heat and then again 3 days later if she is still in a strong heat. If the mare is in a prolonged heat period of 10 days or more, it is best to discontinue breeding her until she has settled down to normal cycles, which will usually occur by the end of March. "If a little is good, a lot is better" does not apply to the breeding of horses; everyday breeding is not a recommended procedure. This often overworks the stallion and increases the chances of establishing an infection in the mare.

Breeding Hygiene

To help prevent the possibility of establishing reproductive tract infections, good breeding hygiene techniques should be used. These include the following procedures:

1. Bandage the tail of the mare—at least the upper 12 to 18 inches, to keep the hair away from the vulva. This also helps avoid the possibility of the cutting of the stallion's penis by these hairs at the time of breeding.
2. Wash the vulva and the rear quarters of the mare that may

EQUINE TEASING AND BREEDING RECORD

Breeder: RODABI-J RANCH—PLEASANT HILL, CA.

MONTH: APRIL   Owner: RODABI-J RANCH

Code: O—Out of Heat; ↑—Coming In; I—In; ↓—Going Out; B—Bred; T—Treated

Mare	1	2	3	4	5	6	7	8	9	10	11	12	13	14	15	16	17	18	19	20	21	22	23	24	25	26	27	28	29	30	31
"RENA"	O	O	O	↑	I	I	B	I	B	I	↓	O	O	O		O		O		O		O		O	O	O	O	O	O		
"CALIE"	O	O	T	O	O	O	O	O	O	O	O	↑	I	I	B	I	B	I	I	B	I	↓	O	O	O		O		O		
"SUESY"	↑	I	B	I	B	I	I	↓	O	O	O		O		O		O		O		O	O	O	↑	I	I	I	B	I	B	I

TEASING and BREEDING SCHEDULE

OPEN UNBRED MARES

(a)   Tease every other day until signs of heat are detected.

(b)   Tease daily while in heat and continue for 2 to 3 days past last signs of her going out.

(c)   Breed on the 2nd and 4th days of heat and only again on the 6th day if mare still shows signs of strong heat.

Note: If in a prolonged heat of 10 days or longer, discontinue breeding until she settles down to normal length (5- to 7-day) heat periods or is examined by a veterinarian.

BRED MARES To Be "TEASED BACK"

(a)   Tease every 2 to 3 days for the 14-day period after last breeding, then tease daily for next 10 days. If no heat is detected during this period, it is a good indication that the mare has conceived.

(b)   After 22 days have passed, tease every 3 to 4 days up to 38 days past last breeding, then tease daily for 7 to 10 days.

(c)   If mare comes back into heat only begin rebreeding schedule on her 3rd day of heat, to avoid force breeding during a "false heat."

Chart II. Teasing and breeding record.

come in contact with the stallion's penis. Use a mild soap (Amway's L.O.C. or Ivory) and rinse well.

3. Wash the stallion's penis before and after breeding.

Restraint

It is always a good practice to use proper restraint on the mare prior to breeding. Even though pasture breeding results in a much higher conception rate, "hand breeding" is a common practice to prevent injury to the stallion. To assure this protection, the mare should be restrained to prevent her kicking the stallion during the breeding procedure. A twitch and a sideline are usually sufficient for this restraint (Fig. 61). Some breeders prefer the use of breeding hobbles as opposed to the sideline. The twitch should be routinely used unless a particular mare is a real twitch fighter and breeds well without it. Such a procedure is a potential danger to the stallion. The twitch (a chain or rope loop placed around the nose and tightened) should always be applied first before any ropes or hobbles are put in place. The twitch should always be the last to be removed after the breeding is completed. This is an important consideration to prevent the possible injury to those mares that badly fight any ropes. A sideline consists of a rope going from a circular rope collar back through a single Dee ring hobble placed below the left fetlock and back again to the collar.

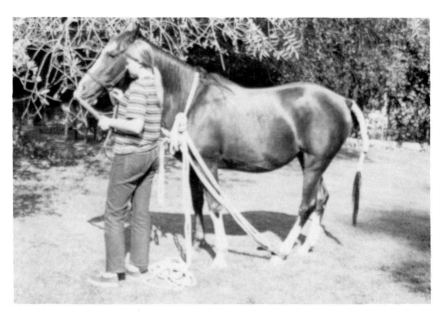

FIG. 61. "Sideline" and twitch used to restrain mare for breeding to prevent injury to stallion (Pat Schwarz).

Just enough slack is taken up in the rope as not to allow the mare to kick back. This does allow her to stand without losing her balance. The sideline is then secured in an easily untied knot. Many different breeding hobbles are available. The least complicated are the best.

Hand-Breeding Procedure

1. Bring the mare out in the open or place her in a well-constructed, safe breeding chute, if one is to be used.
2. Wrap her tail and wash her in preparation for breeding.
3. Bring out the stallion and allow him to get close enough to her to make him become interested and let down his penis. At this time the stallion is taken off to the side—up against a wall or safe fence to wash the penis.
4. Apply the twitch and then either the sideline or breeding hobbles to the mare. (Strapping or tying up a front leg is often a very dangerous procedure and is not recommended.)
5. The stallion may then be allowed to come up to the rear of the mare, approaching her from the left side and held under control by a competent handler. It is a good practice to have a stud shank (chain lead strap) through the left side of the halter over the stallion's nose to the other side of the halter for better control of the animal. It is also advisable to have a 3- or 4-foot quirt in hand if it becomes necessary to use it to control the breeding procedure.
6. If the mare and the stallion are under control and the stallion has developed an erection, he is allowed to mount the mare to complete a cover. If the stallion has a tendency to bite the mare at the time of breeding, padding should be placed over the mare's neck and withers for protection. Flagging of the tail (an up and down movement) of the stallion indicates that a normal ejaculation has occurred.
7. When the stallion desires to dismount (usually after a minute or so), he is allowed to do so, and an attempt should be made to wash his penis at this time. This is often very difficult to do, but is not as important as the prebreeding preparations. He is then returned to his stall or paddock.
8. The ropes are then removed from the mare and the twitch is finally removed. At this time, she is quietly walked around for a few minutes, the tail wrap is removed, and she, too, is returned to her stall or paddock. The practice of throwing cold water on the mare following breeding, in an attempt to prevent her from "throwing out" some of the semen, is not effective and is not a recommended procedure.

Ninth-Day Breeding

This is the breeding of the mare in the first heat period after foaling, usually about the ninth day. The following are pros and cons.

Advantages
1. If a mare is bred at this time, she does have a chance of getting in foal.
2. If a mare does conceive at this breeding, she will foal three weeks earlier the following year. This can be important to those concerned with racing or showing, who want to have bigger foals for competition.
3. A small percentage of mares will show a strong "foaling heat," but will fail to come back in heat again during the breeding season.

Disadvantages
1. Studies have indicated that the usual conception rate for this ninth-day breeding is only 25 to 43% as opposed to 56 to 65% conception rate when mares are bred back on their second heat cycle at approximately 30 days.
2. Abortion rates are approximately 13% as against the 4% considered normal.
3. The rate of dead or diseased foals is 7% as opposed to the less than 1% that is normal.
4. Mares are more susceptible to uterine infections in the first 2 weeks following foaling than at any other time.
5. There is a higher incidence of retained afterbirths and uterine infections following foaling.

Because of the many disadvantages associated with ninth-day breeding, it should not be a routine practice and should only be considered if the mare is examined and found free of vaginal and cervical bruises and is found to be "clean" on cervical culture taken by a veterinarian. Many breeders require a prebreeding veterinary examination and cervical culture on all mares brought in for breeding. This often avoids many problems.

INFERTILITY IN THE MARE

When reviewing the basic physiology of the mare, we see that many physiological and physical changes take place during the estrous cycle. For breeding purposes, four main activities must occur, all at the proper time to ensure conception. These include:
1. The mare must show an apparent heat period so she will be willing to accept the stallion for breeding.
2. She must produce an ovum and develop it to maturity.

3. She must release the ovum (ovulate) at the proper time during her heat period.
4. Her cervix must be relaxed and open at the time of the heat period to allow the entrance of semen at the time of breeding.

Physiological Infertility

There are many variations or deviations from the normal physiological pattern that result in infertility in the mare. These conditions seem to be the predominant causes of infertility in mares of all ages, but especially in older mares and those that have been reproductively inactive for 2 or more years.

1. *Irregular heat cycles* can vary from complete anestrous (no heat) to an excessively prolonged heat period. Frequently, mares not showing an apparent heat period will actually be having "silent heats." These can be picked up by a veterinary examination of the cervix. Prolonged heat periods most often occur early in the breeding season (January through March), but usually correct themselves. This is occasionally due to ovarian disease.
2. *Irregular ovulation* can occur, which may result in the release of the ovum a few days after the heat period and after the death of any sperm that may have been introduced. At times, no ovulation will occur at all as the result of an incomplete development and maturation of the follicle. This can cause a prolonged heat period, as can a tumor of the ovary. These latter two conditions are most common in aged mares.
3. *Incomplete opening of the cervix* is most often the result of reduced hormone activity or from post-foaling cervical scarring.
4. *Chronic aborters* are mares that habitually abort their foals at approximately 60 days. This is the time when the ovary shifts its responsibility of the production of progesterone (a hormone necessary to sustain pregnancy) over to the placenta. Because this transfer is not successfully accomplished, abortion occurs. Because the fetus is so small at this time, there will usually be no other evidence that an abortion has occurred except that the mare comes back into heat. If a mare has been found in foal at least 3 times at 40 days and then found to come back into heat after 60 to 90 days, it can be presumed that she is a chronic aborter. Hormone treatment for this condition should begin as soon as the mare is found in foal and continued up to the last month of pregnancy.
5. *Temporary infertility while nursing* occurs with some mares, as with many women. When this condition is recognized to occur with an individual mare, routine treatment should be

administered prior to her 30-day heat cycle, following foaling, to ensure that her period will be a strong, normal period. This involves the use of a prostaglandin injection or a uterine infusion.

6. *False pregnancy* is the result of a hormonal problem and causes the mare to act and appear in all respects to be in foal. Her heat periods, physically and physiologically, discontinue. This is usually due to a retained corpus luteum that didn't disappear as is normal. If the mare goes full term, she may appear to develop a large abdomen and come into milk. This condition is much more common in the bitch than in the mare. Occasionally the mare may go through the motions of labor, but, of course, produces no foal. Most often these mares again begin to have normal cycles. It is best to catch this condition early and bring the mare back to normal cycles by treatment to avoid losing a whole breeding year.

Fortunately, many of these physiological causes of infertility in the mare respond fairly well to treatment. Many mares with subhormonal activity can be stimulated by the use of prostaglandins or uterine infusions. Prostaglandin is a chemical that dissolves the corpus luteum, usually causing the mare to come back into heat within 10 days; it also causes a pregnant mare to abort. Prostaglandins are commonly used to shorten the periods between heat cycles in mares. Chorionic gonadotrophin is commonly used to help in the development of follicles as well as to assist ovulation. Each individual case should be evaluated by a veterinary examination. It is important that all mares be in good physical condition for breeding.

7. *Hypothyroidism* in the horse is not uncommon and results from a low thyroid-gland activity. It is a condition that is frequently not clinically diagnosed. Mares affected will typically be overweight, have a large heavy crest, and will be very easy keepers. These mares have a tendency to founder, even on grass. Thyroid hormone administration is often necessary to better their chances of conception.

Physical Infertility

1. *Infections* that become established in the uterus of the mare almost always render her unable to conceive or to produce a normal, healthy foal. Such infections are usually caused by bacteria that are normally found in the surrounding environment, but become associated with the reproductive tract through contamination. These infections are not venereal diseases as such, since the causative bacteria are only "op-

portunists" and do not require the tissues of the genital tract for survival.

Studies have shown that nearly 100% of foaling mares pick up a genital tract infection following parturition. Bacteria from the environment are often sucked into the vagina and uterus by the negative pressure created at the time of the expulsion of the foal. Most mares throw off this infection within 7 to 14 days. The natural tissue resistance is surprisingly effective in preventing the establishment of the infection if tissue damage has not been extensive, and the normal healing processes occur without interference.

2. *Contagious equine metritis (CEM)* is a highly contagious bacterial venereal disease of horses that causes an acute purulent (pus-causing) infection of the uterus of the mare. It is a relatively new disease, first identified in England in 1977. The disease has now been found in Ireland, Australia, France, and the United States (Kentucky) and has restricted the movement of horses among these countries. This is one of only two diseases in the horse that are considered venereal diseases. The other is equine coital exanthema, a sporadic herpes virus disease that causes small vesicles (blisters) that heal in 7 to 10 days with no complications.

The bacteria that causes CEM is most often introduced into the mare at the time of breeding, but may be spread by humans. Though the stallion can become infected, it produces no clinical signs, although he often acts as a carrier of the disease. Some mares with no symptoms can become chronic carriers.

When the bacteria infects the lining of the uterus, a thick, sometimes profuse discharge is observed coming from the uterus. Some infections may be limited to just within the vulva so no discharge will be noted. The course of the disease is usually 10 to 14 days in both the treated and untreated mare, but untreated mares often become carriers. Although the bacteria is sensitive to a number of different antibiotics, and although the disease is easily treated in the stallion, treatment of mares is less reliable. Laboratory tests are used to confirm the diagnosis. Incidences of CEM should be reported to the appropriate state and federal authorities.

3. *A retained placenta* (afterbirth) and the breeding of the mare on the ninth day after foaling are the two most predisposing factors in establishing a uterine infection following parturition. The retention of the afterbirth is frequently due to a low-grade, prefoaling infection. Improper nutrition may also be a factor. The foal may or may not be diseased at birth.

When the placenta is retained more than 8 hours veterinary attention should be sought. It should be removed within 24 hours and proper treatment is mandatory to prevent the establishment of an infection and even the possible death of the mare. Deaths following complications of a retained placenta are a frequent occurrence every year.

4. *Pneumovagina* or "wind-sucking" in mares is another predisposing factor to infections. The condition results from the sinking in of the anus, which causes the vulva to be tipped forward and allows air to be sucked into the vagina. This may be due to poor conformation or to poor condition. It is very common in Thoroughbreds. The constant irritation that occurs overcomes tissue resistance and paves the way for infection. Such irritation can also produce an unfavorable chemical reaction with the fluids of the genital tract, thereby shortening the life of the spermatozoa. Artificial insemination in some of these mares is beneficial because it permits by-passing of the local chemical upset if an infection has not already gained a foothold in the uterus. This is especially true with those mares that only suck air while in heat. A fairly simple surgical procedure will usually prevent wind-sucking and may add years of productivity to mares so affected. This surgical procedure is the "Caslick operation," which consists of closing the upper third of the vulva with sutures.

5. The *stallion* can also be a factor in passing infection from one mare to another. This is usually accomplished by mechanical means only. For such passage to occur, it is usually necessary for the stallion to first breed an infected mare, then within 24 hours to breed another mare and introduce this infection into her. Seldom does the stallion himself develop the infection, although this is possible. Mature stallions (over 5 years old) seem very resistant to infections, but young 2-year-olds seem quite susceptible. If a stallion does have an active infection, he doesn't often pass it on to the mares, but this, too, may be possible, though he rarely is able to impregnate a mare when he has an infection.

Some of the other common sources of mechanical contamination that lead to infections are poor breeding hygiene, unsanitary capsuling techniques, the use of unclean vaginal instruments, and the outmoded "horseman's" procedure of "opening up" a mare.

One must bear in mind that not all infections are obvious and vaginal discharge does not always accompany an infection. An infected mare's heat cycle is usually quite regular, but she fails to conceive after repeated breedings. Early abortions (60 to 120 days) may occur in a mare that suddenly comes back into heat after 2 to 4 months of anestrous (no heat). Frequently, no aborted foal is found nor is any discharge noted.

Although infections usually prevent pregnancy, there are some conceptions in which the foal is carried full term, only to be born dead or seriously diseased. Breeding is seldom, if ever, recommended in the case of a known infection.

A cervical or uterine culture is the only technique by which an infection can be diagnosed. Some mares may have a marked discharge that may be only inflammatory with no bacteria present. On the other hand, mares that may appear "clean" may prove to have an extensive infection. The culturing procedure involves taking a sterile sample from the mare's cervix or uterus when she is in full heat and attempting to grow bacteria on a culture medium. If bacteria are present, the diagnosis can be confirmed, and the most effective antibiotics can be selected by running sensitivity tests. Currently, the veterinary profession is taking a second look at the significance of these culture findings.

Minimizing Uterine Infections

1. Use good breeding hygiene.
2. Avoid ninth-day breeding. At no other time is a mare's resistance as low as it is at this time. It often takes 10 to 14 days or longer for a mare to throw off her low-grade post-foaling infection. The uterus has much contracting to do at this time. If ninth-day breeding is felt necessary because of the time factor, have an equine veterinarian give a prebreeding exam and culture.
3. Prior to breeding, culture all mares that have had retained placenta for more than 8 hours, that have had any vaginal discharge, that have been bred through one or more normal heat cycles, but did not conceive (even maiden mares may be infected), or that are unfamiliar or from another stable. Culture any outside mare.

It should be pointed out that infections are difficult to clear up even with extensive and persistent treatment, but become more difficult the longer they go untreated. It is up to the breeder to be aware of this problem and to make every effort to prevent its occurrence by proper management, good breeding hygiene, and routine veterinary assistance.

Infantile uterus is the result of a glandular insufficiency. The ovaries are usually quite small and the uterus is only a fraction of the normal size. These animals occasionally will have enough ovarian development to have heat cycles but will not conceive. This is a cause of permanent sterility with few exceptions. The condition is diagnosed on physical examination by the veterinarian.

Cervical restriction can result from scarring and adhesions that most often occur following a difficult foaling. This condition is difficult to treat effectively and often results in permanent sterility.

INFERTILITY IN THE STALLION

As a rule, infertility in the stallion becomes an evident problem when all or most of the mares bred come back in heat and are not in foal. This is not so evident when the stallion is only breeding a few mares.

Causes

1. *Poor general condition* from inadequate nutrition, parasitism, and disease can impair fertility. Also, mental and physical exhaustion from worrying about breeding, excess use as a teaser, and fence pacing can result in poor sperm quality.
2. *Lack of testicular development* is often a congenital problem but may be the result of early nutritional deficiencies or sickness with a high fever. Occasionally hormonal treatment is effective.
3. *Testicular degeneration* may result from direct injuries or local infections. Treatment for infections may be effective if the damage to the testicles is not extensive.
4. *Masturbation* is a habit that a stallion may develop and is a common cause of lowered fertility. He does this by rubbing the penis up against the abdomen, resulting in an ejaculation. Frequently, this activity is practiced at night and not observed by the owner. Insufficient exercise may predispose to masturbation. The condition is best treated by the use of a plastic stallion ring. This ring is placed on the relaxed penis and fits snugly but not too tight. Frequent examination and care of the ring is necessary to avoid causing damage to the penis.
5. *Improper ejaculation* is a common cause of infertility. This is a condition that occurs when a stallion makes a normal cover but fails to ejaculate, and usually no "flagging" of the tail is observed. The best way to determine that this is occurring is to examine microscopically some of the postbreeding fluids from the penis which are collected as the stallion dismounts. If no sperm is found to be present in this fluid, it is unlikely that the stallion had a normal ejaculation. If this is true, the animal will usually be ready to attempt another cover in just a few minutes and breed again. Occasionally an individual

stallion may make three covers before a normal ejaculation occurs. When this condition is recognized, a postbreeding fluid examination should be made routinely and the mares rebred as necessary. This usually improves the stallion's conception rate immediately.

Semen study can indicate the fertility of a stallion and is used to determine causes of low fertility and sterility. Characteristics of the semen that are noted are color, density, sperm motility, sperm numbers and shapes, and live/dead counts. The fluid is also examined for the presence of pus cells. In addition, the semen can be cultured to determine if there is a bacterial infection. Many stud farms do routine semen studies on their stallions at the beginning of the breeding season and periodic spot checks during the season. Studies show that the normal sperm count of stallions in the winter is about one-half what it is during the spring and summer months.

CHAPTER

7

The Foaling Mare

PREGNANCY

The average gestation period for the mare is 345 days. An easy and fairly accurate method to estimate the foal's due date is to subtract one month from the breeding date and add 10 days (e.g., if the breeding date is May 15, the due date would be April 15 plus 10 days, which would be April 25). A foal born 3 weeks prior to the expected due date will usually show signs of prematurity. Mares carrying normal foals for 13 months are not uncommon.

Riding the Pregnant Mare

A normal, healthy, pregnant mare should be able to be used for most average horse activities up until about the last 8 to 10 weeks. After this time, most mares tire easily. Too much activity can be a significant stress. Jumping, racing, and strenuous rides should be discontinued when the mare is 4 months along. The foal is well protected in the broodmare and it is very difficult to cause an abortion by an outside force, such as a kick. This is especially true during the early months.

Mares that have a repeated history of losing their foals during pregnancy should undergo no forceful activity, especially between 50 and 70 days. This is often a critical time when the hormonal responsibility for maintaining pregnancy is switched over from the ovary to the placenta in the uterus. It is just good common sense not to overexert or stress a pregnant mare.

154

Symptoms of Pregnancy

Mares that are pregnant do not usually come back into heat, although studies have found that about 17% of pregnant mares will show signs of heat. This is more common in mares having their first foal. Usually this "false heat" will be an abnormal period, not lasting much over 24 hours. If breeding of the mare is attempted, she will most often seem receptive up until the last moment, then resist vigorously. It is possible to cause an abortion if the breeding is forced at this time. It is advisable to be certain that the mare is having a seemingly normal heat cycle, by being in heat for at least 3 days before rebreeding.[7]

Tests for Pregnancy

Even though there are laboratory tests to help diagnose pregnancy in the mare, a rectal examination by an experienced equine veterinarian not only is safer, but can be done earlier and usually more accurately and at less expense. This can be done any time after 35 days from being bred.

Ultrasound

Using ultrasound, pregnancy can be detected in the mare at about 18 to 20 days. Twins can be detected and aborted using prostaglandin. The normal incidence of twins is about 8%. This equipment is very expensive and is mostly limited to large animal breeding farm practices.

Embryo Transfer

In cattle it is possible to cause a cow to produce many fertile eggs that can be implanted into donor animals, thus it is possible to get many offspring of highly desirable sires and dams in a given year. At present, breed registries allow only one registration per mare each year; therefore, current interest in embryo transfer is limited. Despite this, we now have on record the delivery of a healthy thoroughbred foal from a surrogate mule.

---

[7]The first "false heat" period most often occurs at the normally predicted time of the next due period—approximately 16 to 18 days later. It is physically impossible for it to be determined that it is a false heat during the short period the mare is "showing in." When examined by a veterinarian, she may show all evidence of being in true heat by having a relaxed cervix and even a follicle developing on an ovary, but still already be pregnant. Since it is necessary for a mare to be approximately 35 days along before a rectal examination by a veterinarian can determine pregnancy, it is wise not to be too anxious to rebreed early in this period. New techniques of determining pregnancy in the mare earlier may change this situation.

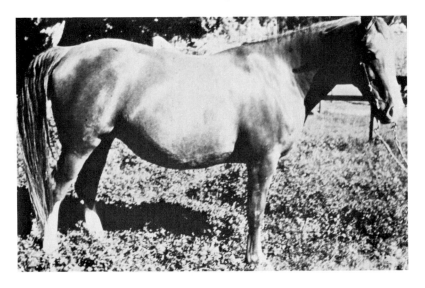

FIG. 62.   Twenty-four hours before foaling. Note enlarged, flattened appearance of abdomen.

Mid-Pregnancy Signs

When the mare is approximately 7 months along, the foal may begin to "drop down," causing the lower abdomen to take on an enlarged, flattened appearance (Fig. 62). From this time on, kicking or movement of the foal may sometimes be observed through the abdominal wall. This is often more evident after the mare has had a drink of cold water. It should be noted that it is not uncommon for some mares to show no outward signs of pregnancy before foaling, while others may look to be very heavy with foal and actually not be pregnant. This latter condition is characteristic of mares going through a false pregnancy.

Eminent Signs That the Foaling Is Near

During the last six weeks, most mares begin to show evidence of "making bag." Some mares may show no evidence of udder development until just before, and on occasion, not until after foaling. The following are the two most consistent signs to indicate that dropping of the foal is very close:

1. "Waxing over" is when the secretion of the first milk is observed on the ends of the teats (Fig. 63). As a rule, approximately 24 hours before foaling, it is first observed as whitish or opaque in color. Within the last 12 hours, it becomes clear, honey-like in color, and may stream out. Though this is the usual sequence of waxing for most mares, some may wax 3 or 4 weeks before foaling and even drip milk, but then dry

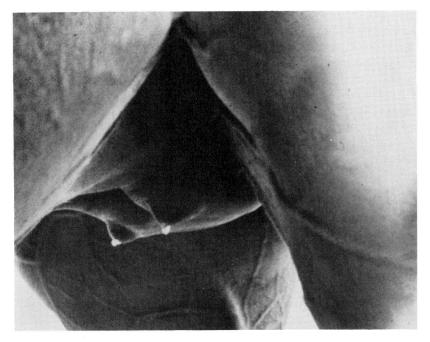

FIG. 63. Mare "waxing over" just 24 hours before foaling.

up again. Others, usually maiden mares, may show no signs of waxing before delivery.
2. "Relaxing of the vulva" does not noticeably occur until the last 12 to 18 hours. The vulva then appears very relaxed and elongated. This is probably the most consistent sign that foaling is near.

Preparing for Foaling

It should be the concern and duty of every owner of a pregnant mare to provide a safe location in which she can foal.

It is best to allow the mare to foal in an area away from other horses. Very commonly, other mares will try to steal a new foal from its mother, which can result in much distress to the mare and possible injury to the newborn foal. Not uncommonly, other horses will attack a newborn and kill it if the mother is unable to protect it (Fig. 64). This can be a very difficult, even impossible, problem if more than one horse is trying to reach the foal. After a foal is born—away from other horses—it is a good policy not to attempt to put the mare and foal out with other horses until the foal is at least 2 or 3 weeks old. Then it is best if the other horses can first have a chance to become acquainted with the newcomer over a fence. Allowing mares to foal out in a pasture with other pregnant mares is a common practice, but close supervision should be the rule.

The foaling area should be safe. If the mare is allowed to foal out in a pasture or range, there should be no steep hillsides, ravines, or steeply banked stream beds in the area. Many newborn foals die as a result of falls in uneven and unsafe foaling areas.

The fence around the foaling area should be safe and low. Barbed wire is never safe, especially around newborn foals. The fence should not have a large space under it. If it does, the space should be secured with a safe stock wire fence or board close to the ground. This is necessary because a new foal can easily roll out under such a fence and get into an area with other horses or fall into an area where it may be injured. If the foal does get in with other horses, it may very well try to nurse from any one of them, including any gelding that might be there. This is true because it usually takes several days for it to be certain who its mother is. Too frequently, other horses will take this opportunity to attack this new foal, and the results are often disastrous.

Probably the best area for foaling is a well-fenced, clean, green pasture, but here, too, mares should be closely observed during the foaling process so that problems can be prevented or dealt with quickly if they occur.

Foaling in a stall has two major advantages: it can provide

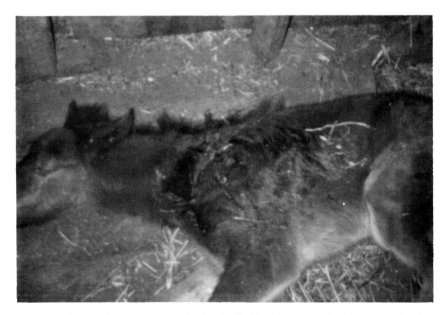

FIG. 64. Newborn foal that was attacked and killed by other horses in the pasture with the foaling mare. Mares should always be allowed to foal away from other horses.

protection from bad weather and other animals; and it makes close supervision possible and allows for immediate help if such is required. Fortunately, most mares foal with no trouble or complications, but it is best to be prepared when help is needed. A foaling stall should be large—at least 12 × 12 feet for small horses, but 14 × 14 feet or *larger* is better. A double stall is ideal. If no stall is available, then a clean paddock or corral at least 30 × 30 feet should be provided. This much space is required to allow the mare to protect her foal from other horses hanging over the fence.

Bedding of the foaling stall should be good, clean straw, which should be slightly dampened if it is at all dusty. Deep bedding is recommended. Shavings and all dusty bedding should be avoided to prevent possible introduction of infection into the mare shortly after foaling. Just following the forceful expulsion of the foal, there is an instant of negative pressure that can suck in dust and bacteria from the surroundings. Also, the post-foaling membranes that are still protruding from the vulva often become contaminated, introducing infection when they move back into the vulva.

Supplies

It is wise to have the following materials immediately available at the foaling barn: warm water, soap, roll of cotton, clean buckets, clean tail bandage (e.g., 4-inch gauze roll), clean towels, tincture of iodine or other navel antiseptic, umbilical tape or semiheavy string, a pair of scissors, aspirin, materials for a bran mash, a pail or other container for the afterbirth, and an enema can with a soft rubber hose for the foal.

If the mare clearly indicates she is very close to foaling, it is desirable to wrap her tail and wash her vulva and buttock area. The udder should also be washed and dried, paying attention to cleaning out the material accumulated between her teats. Then it is best to leave her alone, remaining out of the stall and maintaining a careful watch.

Prefoaling Colic

It is not uncommon for a mare to develop signs of abdominal distress, such as sweating, looking around at her abdomen, and appearing to be in pain. This can occur as early as 6 weeks prior to foaling or any time up to when she is due. Early uterine contractions, preparing for the foaling process, are considered to be the cause. Specific antispasmodic and analgesic (for pain) drugs will alleviate these signs. Hot bran mash with aspirin is also often effective. The onset of an abortion has to be considered as another possible cause for these symptoms, but lying down and straining as if in labor are more specific signs of an impending abortion.

BIRTH OF THE FOAL

About 90% of the time, mares foal at night. Because they have very strong abdominal muscles, the foaling process only takes about 15 to 30 minutes. If a mare is in hard labor (bearing down and obviously pressing to deliver the foal) for more than 30 minutes, immediate professional or experienced help is required. Do not rush the mare. Allow her time for an unassisted delivery if all seems to be going normally. Usually, just prior to going into hard labor, the mare will appear nervous, eat small amounts of feed, and then walk around. Some pawing at the ground, lightly kicking at the abdomen, frequent passing of small amounts of manure, lying down and getting up at short intervals are all common signs that the foaling is close at hand.

Shortly after the "breaking of the water bag" around the foal, hard labor begins and a "bubble" appears through the vulva (Fig. 65). Most mares foal lying down. The normal presentation is the two front feet appearing fairly evenly together, followed shortly by the nose and the head just behind the knees. Once the front legs and head are out, the foal is usually expelled quickly with great force.

TIMES FOR ASSISTANCE

Most normal mares require little or no assistance. Difficult births are usually due to weak, diseased, or dead foals that are not in the normal positions for foaling (Fig. 66). Because the normal delivery period is so short and occurs under great pressure, it is advisable for the owner or attendant to be familiar with the method and procedure of correcting situations that require immediate attention. Professional help should always be sought for foaling cases where hard labor has been going on for more than 30 minutes. In cases of prolonged labor with no appearance of the foal or where it is evident that marked abnormal presentation is the problem, the mare should be walked slowly until the veterinarian arrives. This discourages straining and lessens the chances of injury to the mare or the foal.

All procedures in assisting the foaling mare should be done with clean hands and under conditions that are as antiseptic as possible. The tail should be wrapped and the genital area should be washed.

The following are the most common types of abnormal foal presentations which result in difficult births (dystochias). Their descriptions and the procedures outlined are to acquaint the owner with these problems so that he may be able to help a mare when needed. Some procedures are simple, whereas others are

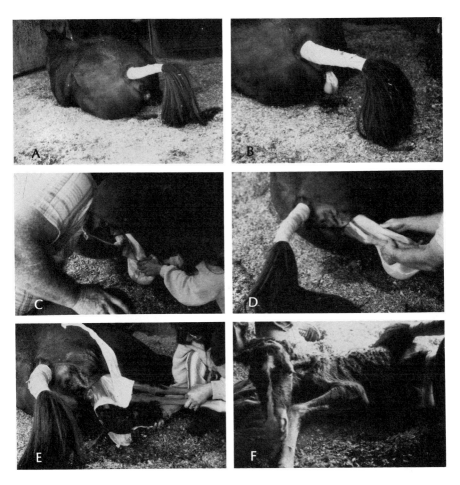

FIG. 65. Birth of the foal. (Jones, W.E.: Genetics and Horse Breeding. Lea & Febiger, Philadelphia, 1982.)

more involved. It should be emphasized that these more involved procedures should only be attempted in cases of true emergencies or when professional help is not immediately available.

Mare Attempts Foaling While Standing

Signs. The mare will begin to produce the foal while standing and then proceed to walk around with the partially delivered foal.

Procedure. Since nothing can induce a mare to lie down, it is best to control her head with a halter and to not allow her to rub up against the stall wall or purposely press up against the partially delivered foal. As soon as the foal is about to be delivered, it should be helped to the floor without being dropped.

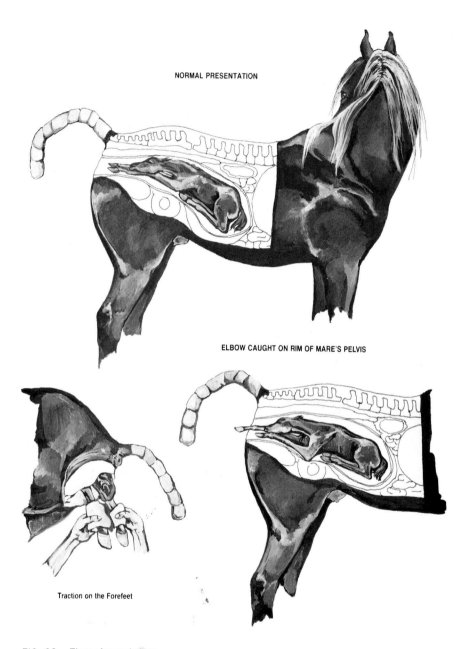

NORMAL PRESENTATION

ELBOW CAUGHT ON RIM OF MARE'S PELVIS

Traction on the Forefeet

FIG. 66.   Times for assistance.

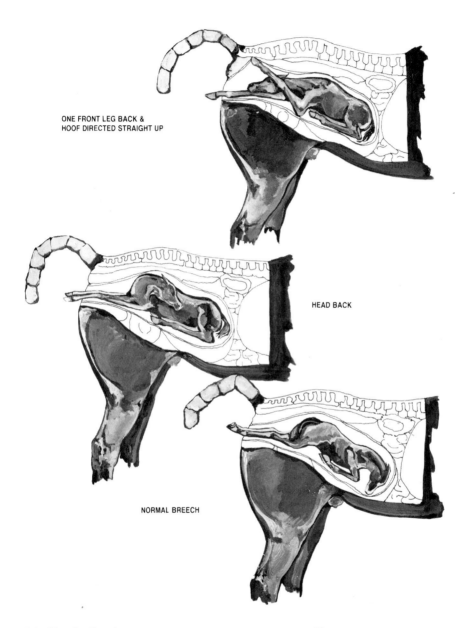

FIG. 66.   Continued

Elbow Caught on Rim of Mare's Pelvis

Signs. The front feet will not appear together, one being back a short distance within the vulva.

Procedure. The hand is inserted into the vagina where the foot is grasped and gently pulled out to a position even with the other foot. No ropes or chains are used. Easy pulling on the legs in a downward arc can assist the mare in the final delivery, but this is not usually necessary.

One Front Leg Back

Signs. Only one foot and leg appear followed by the muzzle of the foal slightly protruding from the vulva.

Procedure. The head and thus the body is pushed back down into the uterus to make room to pass the hand and arm into the vagina. The end of the hoof is sought, and is brought on around into normal position and pulled up even with the other foot. The end of the hoof is cupped in the hand while bringing it around in order to prevent injury to the wall of the uterus. Normal delivery should follow.

One Front Leg Back and Hoof Directed Straight Up

Signs. Outwardly, it appears that just one leg is back or the elbow is possibly caught on the rim of the mare's pelvis. A slight bulging out of the anus and surrounding tissue during periods of bearing down gives one a clue to this problem. One is made aware of the situation as soon as the leg is sought within the vagina. When this condition is suspected, immediate action is indicated.

Procedure. Same as for one leg back (i.e., cup end of hoof with hand and bring leg down into normal position).[8]

Head Back

Signs. Both front legs well extended out through the vulva with no head appearing slightly behind the knees as would be normal.

Procedure. The body is pushed back down into the uterus while an attempt is made to cup the hand over the foal's muzzle and pull the head around into normal position. The description is much easier than the procedure. Patience and care are needed for

[8]If this condition is not discovered very early and corrected, the strong pressure of labor contractions forces the foot straight up through the upper vaginal wall, into the rectum, and out through the anus. This severe laceration then allows manure to drop into the vaginal cavity. Extensive surgery is necessary to repair this condition and the mare's potential use for future breeding may be permanently affected.

success with no injury to the mare. Always be firm but gentle. Once the head is brought out, normal delivery should follow.

Hip Lock

Signs. The mare seems to be having difficulty after the foal's head and shoulders appear.

Procedure. The front legs are grasped with the hands and the foal is gently rotated almost 180 degrees while being gently but firmly pulled downward toward the mare's hocks. The foal then is rotated back again almost 180 degrees applying pressure in the same direction. This will help "unscrew" the foal's hips through the mare's pelvis. The principle is similar to that of taking a chair through a narrow doorway.

Normal Breech—Back Legs First

Signs. When the feet protrude from the vulva, it will be noted that the soles of the hooves are facing up and not down as is normal. To investigate the situation, the hand is passed into the vagina and the first joint up from the fetlock is examined to determine whether it is a hock or a knee. The hock joint is very pointed; the web of the hock is prominent and when the joint is bent (flexed) the fronts of the hooves move in the direction of the bend. The knee joint is rounded and, when bent, the heels of the hooves move in the direction of the bend.

Procedure. The feet are grasped with the hands, with or without a towel, and gentle but firm pressure is exerted, pulling evenly in the direction of the mare's hocks. This help should be coordinated with the mare's pushing efforts. It is not necessary to turn the foal all the way around before delivery. Prompt delivery is important because a breech presentation can result in a premature breaking of the umbilical cord within the birth canal, which causes a cutting off of the oxygen supply to the foal. The newborn foal should be vigorously massaged while being dried to encourage normal breathing as soon as possible.

THE AFTERBIRTH

After the foal is born, the afterbirth, or placenta, is usually passed within a few minutes, but may be retained for several hours. If it is not passed, a knot tied in it (the use of gauze or a strip of cloth is helpful to tie it up in a knot) will give it added weight, which may help it to pass. Do not try to pull it free by force, which may cause some of it to tear loose inside or cause the whole uterus to prolapse (turn inside out). Either of these conditions can cause severe complications such as acute uterine infection, founder, or even death. If the placenta is not passed within 8 hours, a veterinarian should be called so that it can be definitely removed within 24 hours.

POST-FOALING UTERINE CRAMPS

It is not uncommon for mares to show evidence of colicky pains shortly after delivery of the foal. This is even more common in mares that do not pass the placenta right away.

The mare will frequently want to remain lying down and may look back at her flank. A cold sweat and quivering are not uncommon signs. After she gets up, she still appears uneasy and may squeal if the foal attempts to nurse. These signs usually last 10 to 30 minutes and will often pass without specific treatment. The immediate offering of a hot bran mash in which 10 aspirins are dissolved (5-grain human size) will provide some distraction or relief. Occasionally, use of a specific antispasmodic and analgesic is used by the veterinarian to relieve this condition. This condition can delay the mare's interest in her foal and perhaps cause her to neglect it when it might need her attention (e.g., to remove persistent membranes from the face of the foal).

POST-FOALING INTRA-ABDOMINAL BLEEDING

This is not an uncommon complication to what appeared to be a normal foaling or a difficult birth. The condition most often results from the rupture of the large blood vessels within the large ligament (the middle uterine ligament) that supports the uterus. At first, the bleeding is restricted and retained within the tissues of the ligament. If no further rupturing of this ligament occurs, the mare will survive. Most often within hours or up to 2 or 3 days post-foaling, the tissues of the ligament do break, releasing the previously restricted blood. The massive bleeding that results will cause the death of the mare. This condition can occur in a mare at any age.

The mare may or may not show any symptoms prior to going into sudden shock and death. If symptoms occur right away, she may stay down after foaling and develop an overall coldness to her body, including her ears. She may show facial signs of anxiety. There may be acute colicky signs, which are shortly followed by death. Cold ears is the most common indication that this condition is present when accompanied by the other signs described.

No treatment is effective for this condition because the blood vessel damage is too large to treat before the massive bleeding causes death in the animal. If the condition is believed to have occurred in a surviving mare, careful examination may verify this, although stall rest for 4 weeks is probably the best treatment (without the examination).

8

Care of the Foal and Post-Foaling Mare

FIRST CARE OF THE NEWBORN FOAL

Once the foal arrives, it is important that it begin to breathe promptly. If necessary, any membrane or fluids from the foal's nostrils and mouth should be removed with a towel. Brisk massaging of the chest and body with towels stimulates normal breathing. If a large amount of fluid seems to be obstructing breathing, the foal can be lifted up by his hind legs and swung in pendulum fashion, which allows the flow of fluids out of the respiratory passages. Though this is a real project with large foals, it is worth the effort to clear the respiratory tract and stimulate normal breathing. Few foals need any assistance, but prompt action can save the life of a foal that needs this help.

Attention is then directed to the navel cord. If the navel cord does not break away immediately, allow it to remain intact for as long as 5 minutes, or until it stops pulsating. The foal may receive a significant amount of extra blood from the mare at this time. Never just cut the cord as this may cause excessive bleeding. If the cord does not break away normally because it appears very dry and fibrous, tie it off at the indented area about $1\frac{1}{4}$ to 2 inches from the body wall of the foal using a disinfected ligature (string soaked in iodine). Then cut the cord. Always soak the stump of the navel cord of the newborn foal as soon as possible in a suitable disinfectant (tincture of iodine is commonly used). This procedure is to prevent the entrance of bacteria and serious infection into the foal's body through the navel cord.

In addition to the treatment of the navel cord, it has been shown that the administration of antibiotics within the first 24 to 48 hours after birth has reduced 90% of the cases of navel ill and other serious infections of newborn foals. This procedure—along with giving tetanus antitoxin and a vitamin A, D, and B-complex injection—is now routine and is highly recommended as a segment of Equine Preventative Medicine Techniques.

THE FIRST MILK

During the first 24 hours after birth, the newborn foal is capable of absorbing whole protein from the digestive tract. (Recent studies indicate that this may only be true for the first 12 hours.) This makes it possible for it to take in antibodies from the mare's first milk, which is called *colostrum.* These antibodies give the foal a high degree of immunity against many common bacterial infections. It is therefore very important that a newborn foal receive this colostrum.

ASSISTING THE FIRST NURSING

The first nursing will normally occur within a period from 15 minutes to 2 hours after birth. If the foal has not been up or attempted to nurse by this time, it is advisable to help the foal to find the nipples and get its first milk. The need for this assistance may be due to one of several reasons: weakening from premature birth or disease; early post-foaling injury; or a reluctant mother not allowing the foal to nurse.

Procedure

1. The mare should be haltered and held at the head by an assistant. The first nursing is a painful experience for the mare because the same hormone that causes "milk let down" also stimulates the uterus to contract, thus starting it to return to its normal size and state of health. Because the uterus and birth canal have just experienced quite a bit of stretching and trauma, these contractions are painful.[9]

---

[9]To give the mare relief from the normal pain shortly after foaling and to make it less painful for her to pass manure, a bran mash with 10 aspirins is offered to her very shortly after the foaling process is completed or at her normal feeding period. The use of a twitch and/or a tranquilizer may be necessary for mares that are reluctant to accept their foal. This is common in mares with their first foal. Twitching the mare and forcing her to allow the foal to nurse may be necessary several times the first day. As the pain of nursing subsides and the mare gets more used to the foal she usually accepts her maternal responsibilities.

2. The udder should be washed and dried; the material collected between the teats should be cleaned out.
3. The foal is then guided back to the flank area. The udder is gently massaged for a minute or two and a little milk is squirted out of each teat to stimulate "milk let down."
4. With some of this first milk, which is very sweet and sticky on the hands and fingers, the foal is allowed to nurse a finger and thus be led in close to the nipples. It is normal for the foal to want to butt up to feel pressure on his head while it is in seeking the nipples. While one hand directs the foal back to the nipples, the other hand is placed over its forehead so that it can feel this head pressure. This helps to retain its attention longer during its efforts to find its first meal.
5. If the foal is over 5 hours old and has not learned to nurse, it is advisable that continued attempts in assisting it be made every 30 to 60 minutes until it catches on.

INSUFFICIENT MILK

Many times mares will foal with little or no "bag," and it seems that the foal is continuously nursing in efforts to satisfy its hunger. Very often, this stimulation alone will cause the mare to come into milk within a day or two to meet the foal's requirements. Occasionally, hormones are helpful for this. The use of a tranquilizer is very helpful to increase milk production in a nervous horse. Since it is normal for a foal to nurse very frequently (about every 10 to 15 minutes), it will keep the udder nursed down. One way to get an idea of a mare's milk production is to keep the foal from nursing for about 2 hours to see how much the udder fills and becomes enlarged.

THE NECESSITY FOR MILK SUPPLEMENT FOR THE FOAL

Supplementing the milk received from normal nursing may be indicated if: the foal is constantly attempting to nurse but appears to swallow very little if anything, if the mare's udder shows very little development, if the foal shows no apparent filling out after a few days, or if the mare's udder does not fill markedly when the foal is kept from nursing for 1 to 2 hours.

If a milk supplement is to be given, either a Coke bottle or a lamb's milk bottle fitted with a lamb's nipple is a satisfactory container for this purpose. A warmed milk substitute works well, such as Foal Lac (Borden's), Suckle (Albers), or the following formula for orphan foals: 20 ounces of milk, 12 ounces of water, and 4 tablespoons of Karo syrup. When feeding a foal from a bottle, it is important that the foal be either standing or lying straight up on its chest. Milk forced down, especially if the foal is lying on its side, is likely to enter the lungs. These foals should be taught to drink from a bucket and eat grain as soon as possible.

DISEASES OF THE NEWBORN FOAL

Constipation

Constipation is not an uncommon problem in the newborn foal. At birth, it is normal for the digestive tract of the foal to contain a black, usually firm fecal material called meconium. Occasionally, the first manure is too firm for normal passage.

Signs. The foal will show evidence of constipation by frequently lifting its tail and straining. This straining is often followed by vigorous swishing of the tail. Once the foal has had a chance to nurse the mare, the resulting manure can be identified by its being yellowish in color and somewhat soft.

Procedure. To relieve the constipation, a mild enema is indicated. One to two pints of warm, soapy water can be given using an enema can or funnel through a soft rubber tube, directed about 2 to 4 inches into the rectum. Never direct a metal-tipped syringe into the rectum for this purpose (accidental penetration of the intestinal wall is possible). Allow the enema water to flow by gravity rather than by forcing in under pressure. The constipation is frequently caused by a local blockage just inside the anus. If one is careful, this firm mass can often be removed with a finger. Extreme care should be the rule to prevent injury to the rectal tissue. An enema properly given is the safest procedure. Fleets enemas are effective and convenient.

Meconium Impaction

Occasionally, a large ball of the first manure will be retained in part of the intestinal tract and be too far forward to be reached by an enema.

Signs. The foal may appear constipated, but symptoms of acute colic (getting up and down, rolling, and sweating) will be accompanied by the foal's periodic standing up and straining to pass manure.

Treatment. Such cases should receive veterinary attention as soon as possible. Often it is necessary to administer a sedative and effective analgesic to keep the foal from injuring itself. This medication, along with a fairly large dose (12 to 16 ounces) of milk of magnesia or other suitable cathartic given by way of a stomach tube, will often relieve this condition. Fluids and antibiotics may have to be given for the treatment of secondary shock and stress.

Diarrhea

Signs. Diarrhea in the foal can be the result of many different causes, which include: (1) the mare's producing excessive amount of milk; (2) generalized diseases; (3) local intestinal infections or inflammation (enteritis), which may result from the foal's eating its mother's manure; and (4) possible intestinal parasites that were already picked up early in these first few days of life.

"Ninth day diarrhea" in the foal is commonly seen when the mare comes into her first heat period following foaling. It had been thought that the mare's hormones affected her milk, which then in turn caused diarrhea in the foal, but research indicates rather that it may be the result of very early intestinal infestation of blood worms. More work needs to be done to substantiate these findings.

Procedure. If the diarrhea is relatively mild, the foal will often recover on its own, untreated, in 1 or 2 days. Heavy-milk-producing mares should have their grain reduced until the foal no longer has diarrhea. The administration of Kaolin-Pectate (1 to 2 ounces) twice a day for 1 to 2 days is often effective. This can be given with a large (35 ml) disposable syringe, a turkey basting syringe, or a tablespoon (2 tablespoons equal 1 ounce) administered into the corner of the mouth while the foal is backed into a corner.

If the diarrhea shows very watery to straight water or any evidence that it is causing the foal to stop eating (mare's udder will be filled and possibly dripping milk), or if the foal seems sick and depressed, very early veterinary attention should be sought. Broad-spectrum antibiotics, steroids, and fluid therapy are often necessary to save such foals. (Oxytetracycline I.V. works very well.)

Navel Ill

Navel ill is usually a fatal disease in newborn foals. It is caused by a bacterial infection contracted through contamination of the umbilical cord soon after birth and sometimes prenatally from an infected uterus. There are a number of different bacteria involved in this serious disease. Commonly, the infection enters the blood stream through the umbilical cord and spreads to the liver, the joints, and throughout the body, causing a generalized infection and death.

Signs. At first the foal appears depressed and weak and will not nurse. The best indication of a foal's not eating is the swelling up of the mare's udder and the dripping of milk. Death may occur within 24 hours, or the foal may seem perfectly normal for the first 12 to 14 days, but then develop the "joint ill" form of this

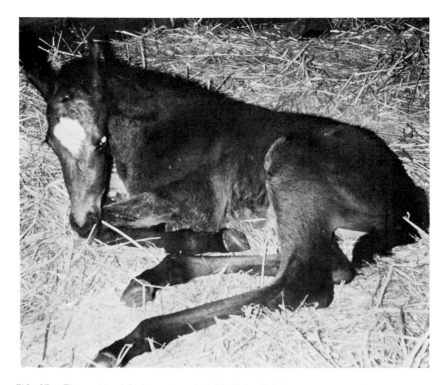

FIG. 67.   Thoroughbred foal ten days old with "joint ill." The stud fee was $5,000.00 and the foal died as a result of the infection. Routine use of antibiotics in newborn foals will almost always prevent this problem.

disease (Fig. 67). Stiffness, enlarged joints, and inability to walk or stand are signs of joint involvement. The animal may succumb shortly after the symptoms occur, or may linger on for as long as three weeks. Animals that recover are rarely completely normal again.

Procedure. Since medical treatment is most often unsuccessful, prevention is important. This mainly involves good management, which includes providing a sanitary environment for foaling, applying a suitable disinfectant (such as tincture of iodine) to the navel shortly after the foal is born, and routine administration of antibiotics to the newborn foal within 24 to 48 hours after birth. Veterinary attention at this time is also helpful in preventing other post-foaling disease problems.

Ruptured Bladder

A foal born with a ruptured bladder is not uncommon. The exact cause is not certain, but it is most likely the result of the pressure exerted on the foal as it passes through the birth canal.

If the foal has a full bladder at this time and if it is extra large or received extra pressure from the mare, it is conceivable that such a rupture could occur. This condition seems to occur more often in stud colts than in fillies.

Signs. At birth, the foal usually appears quite normal. After about 12 hours, it may be noticed to be less alert and seem a little dull. He may show evidence of constipation, but the symptom of being less alert does not disappear after it passes manure. Straining to urinate with the passage of little or no urine can be a very significant clue to the problem. It should be noted that if the tear in the bladder happens to be small and high on the bladder wall, it will be possible for the foal to pass some urine when it attempts to do so. Do not eliminate the possibility of ruptured bladder if some urine seems to be passed normally. Around the third day, the abdomen will begin to bulge as if the foal were bloated. At this time, it is becoming very toxic and lethargic and lies around even more than normal, losing interest in nursing (Fig. 68). The mare's udder may be distended and dropping milk, which would give evidence of the foal's not eating. Owners should always look for this sign when caring for a new foal. Mild colic signs of slight kicking at the abdomen and uneasiness may also be seen.

The diagnosis is suspected by the veterinarian when he sees a foal with this distended abdomen and a history of the other symptoms just discussed. The diagnosis is made when he taps (punc-

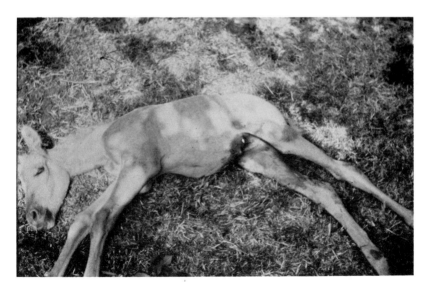

FIG. 68.   Foal with ruptured bladder. Foal became lethargic and developed distended abdomen in first two to three days of life.

tures) the abdominal wall with a large-gauge needle and gets a free flow of urine from the body cavity. Early diagnosis is essential for treatment to be successful.

Procedure. Prompt surgery to repair the bladder is needed, along with good supportive therapy of fluids and antibiotics. If the rupture has occurred within the bony pelvis, the surgery is impossible and the foal is best put to sleep because death is certain.

Pneumonia

Pneumonia in young animals is a serious disease problem, but this is even more true in foals under 30 days of age. It is most often a complication of an upper respiratory tract infection that is not treated or undertreated. Although streptococcus bacteria have been most often the cause, more recently corynebacterium bacteria have been causing major outbreaks on some breeding farms. This is the same bacterium that causes chronic abscesses in horses. Pneumonia caused by this bacterium most often has a fatal outcome. Pneumonia is the most common condition that results in death in Arabian foals born with combined immunodeficiency (CID).

Signs. The foal may develop a cough and have a runny nose. The temperature will usually go up to between 103 and 106 degrees. Marked reduction in appetite is noticed and the foal will begin to be observed having difficulty breathing. This is one strong argument against trying to have mares foal in January, unless one is well equipped to care properly for these animals under winter conditions.

Procedure. A very diligent antibiotic therapy program should be instigated. This program should be extended over a minimum period of 10 to 14 days. If only haphazard treatment is given or if treatment is discontinued too soon, the foal has a great tendency to relapse and be much worse off and less able to respond favorably. Fluids should not be given intravenously because they have a tendency to aggravate and worsen the congestion in the lungs. Good nursing is indicated (e.g., keep in warm, draft-free stall, use heat lamps, and try to encourage a good appetite by treating the foal with aspirin and decongestant to make it feel better). Owners should follow the directions of the attending veterinarian very closely. Pneumonia is a very serious problem and such cases should always be under the care of a veterinarian.

Combined Immunodeficiency (CID)

This is a genetic disorder of foals of Arabian breeding in which there is a lack of two important types of white blood cells (T and B lymphocytes) which protect them from infection. The disease is characterized by signs of pneumonia, intermittent fever, diarrhea, and a fatal outcome (100%).

Cause. CID is a recessive trait that must be passed by both sire and dam. If carrier parents are bred, there is one chance in four of producing a CID foal, two chances in four of producing a carrier foal, and one chance in four of being normal. There is no test for carriers. The disease has been diagnosed in non-purebreds, but all have had Arabian breeding. This disease has not been observed in any other breed. Based on surveys done in Colorado and in Australia, the number of foals affected seems to be between 2% and 3%. It is felt that the disease is currently carried by 26% of Arabian mares and stallions. There is a similar disease that affects human babies. There is no connection with the disease known as AIDS (acquired immunodeficiency syndrome) that has recently been reported in epidemic numbers in the U.S. and other countries.

The missing lymphocytes make the foals highly susceptible to secondary infections such as adenoviral bronchopneumonia and diarrhea-causing agents.

Symptoms. A thick nasal and ocular discharge is first noticed. This is followed by coughing and difficulty breathing as pneumonia develops. The body temperature may vary from normal to 106 degrees. Symptoms may occur as early as 2 weeks of age or as late as 5 months. Most affected foals develop symptoms before they are 8 weeks of age and inevitably die.

Diagnosis. The symptoms can look and be similar to those seen in foals of any breeding that did not receive enough passive immunity passed from the colostrum. Laboratory findings can be used to make the CID diagnosis. Foals with a lymphocyte count of less than 1000 per mm^3 of blood should be considered suspect.

If one is truly interested in reducing the incidence of this disease, then the breeding of known carriers should be avoided.

Nursing and First Aid. Sick foals with respiratory tract infections are treated with antibiotics and cough medication, and provided with draft-free shelter. Heat lamps are also beneficial. Even though bone marrow transplants have been effective in the treatment of this disease in human babies, no suitable compatible donors have been found in horses. The disease is 100% fatal.

Weak or Crooked Legs of the Newborn Foal

The birth of foals with weak tendons, contracted tendons, or crooked legs such as "knock-kneed," "calf-kneed" (bent backwards), "over on the knees," and wobbly hocks are not uncommon (Figs. 69 and 70).

Cause. The exact causes of these conditions have not been

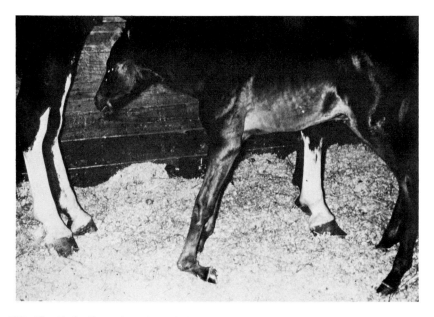

FIG. 69.   Foal with weak tendons. Splints were used to give support. Many foals are born with weak legs that correct themselves within the first seven to fourteen days.

clearly established. It is commonly thought that improper nutrition in the pregnant mare and genetic factors are possible causes.

Treatment. The specific treatment will vary according to the condition and the severity of that condition. It should be stated that the author feels that too often these conditions are overtreated. He has observed that many foals that look like "pretzels" at birth miraculously straighten themselves within 10 to 21 days with no treatment. The author does give credit to vitamin A injections for the improvement of these conditions, especially in the case of contracted tendons.

It should be kept in mind that the skin over the legs of young foals is *very fragile* and is easily affected by pressure necrosis (pressure sores from bandages). The resulting wounds often leave permanent scars. Because of this, the author believes in being very conservative in deciding to apply braces or bandages to the legs of these foals. The main indications for them are the foal's inability to stand and nurse without them and the scraping of the front of an overflexed pastern or ankle joint.

Foals with the so-called "knock-kneed" condition can be treated by the use of a gunny sack roll supported between the front legs (Fig. 71). More serious cases may require such treatment as epiphyseal stapling to straighten the legs. Consult your veterinarian for specific advice and treatment.

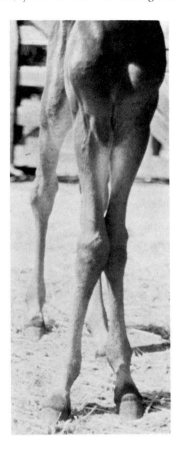

FIG. 70.   Foal born with "knock knees."

A recently developed minor surgical procedure has proven very effective in correcting some congenital angular deformities. The procedure is called "periosteal transection." The technique is used to stimulate bone growth on the concave side of the deformity. It has many advantages over epiphyseal stapling and the screws and wires that were once used to control bone growth.

TURNING OUT MARES AND FOALS

It is best to keep a mare and foal stalled for the first 12 to 24 hours to allow the foal to learn how to nurse and to get acquainted with its mother. It will often take several days before a foal learns who its mother is. This period is sometimes needed for the mare to get over her initial pain and resentment toward the foal before her protective instincts take effect. Weather conditions should always be considered before new foals are exposed to the outside world. Some shelter is always advisable.

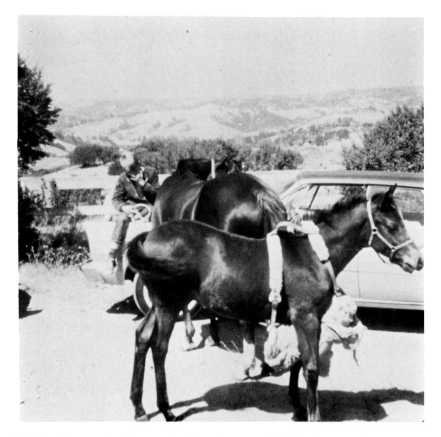

FIG. 71.   Gunny sack roll was used to force knees apart while foal was growing.

Mares with new foals should be kept by themselves for about 3 weeks in a paddock or pasture area before they are placed out with other horses. It is best, also, to allow the other horses to meet and become familiar with the newcomer over a fence for at least 1 to 3 weeks before they are put together. If very new foals must be out with other horses, a large area should be provided and close supervision is essential to prevent aggressive horses from causing injuries.

Early exercise out of a stall will assist the envolution (return to normal) of the uterus. Mares that had problems or that don't appear completely normal should not be rushed outside. It is also important that the foal be vigorous and nursing well before being turned out. This exercise will help the mare to rid herself of the accumulated debris in the uterus. It should be noted that it is normal for mares to pass a large amount of *chocolate-colored post-foaling discharge* on or about the fifth or sixth day. This normally passes over a short period of time and leaves the genital tract clean and healthy in appearance. It is a normal hygienic process. A persistent thick vaginal discharge should be brought to the attention of a veterinarian (it may indicate an infection).

RIDING THE NURSING MARE

As a rule, it is best not to begin to ride the mare for the first 3 weeks following foaling. She should have this time to adjust to caring for her foal. After this time, the mare might be used for short 10- to 15-minute periods of light work. The first few times the mare is taken out of sight of the foal should be very short periods (5 to 10 minutes). It is important that the foal be secured behind a good fence at this time. These periods can gradually be increased so that by the time the foal is 6 to 8 weeks old, the riding periods may be stretched to half-hours. Prolonged riding periods of 2 hours or more are not recommended until the foal is at least 4 to 5 months old. Many mares will begin to normally drop off in milk production near the fifth month of lactation, at which time longer periods away from the foal are not so stressful and painful. Riding a mare with a full udder at the peak of her milk production can be very painful for the mare and can reduce her milk production.[10]

A mare whose udder seems very congested after a ride can be treated with 50 grains of aspirin in her grain. This will help very much to reduce the swelling and discomfort.

WEANING THE FOAL

One the average, most foals are weaned between the ages of 5 and 6 months. Foals in good condition or foals nursing from a mare that is losing flesh can be weaned at 4 months of age with no harmful effects. This is especially true if the foal is already eating hay and grain well and is on a conscientious worming program.

Much is often made of the necessity of having the mare and foal out of sight and out of hearing of each other. This is not essential and the author feels that such complete separation even adds to the stress of the situation. Foals can be weaned very successfully just by separating them from their mothers by a good fence. The fact that this fence be good and safe is important; either a high chain-linked fence or a good board electric fence can be quite satisfactory. The foals seem less concerned about their moth-

---

[10]It is the back pressure on the milk-producing glands that stops further production.

ers being on the other side of a fence than they do by having them completely gone.

It is always a good idea to cut down almost completely on the mare's grain for about 5 days before the weaning is begun. On a given day, the mares and foals are separated by the fence. It is always best to move the mare to the new location. It is also good practice to have young foals become acquainted and be together with gentle geldings or unbred mares before weaning time. They make very good babysitters when the day comes when their mothers are not immediately available. Foals usually need to be kept separated from their mothers for 6 weeks for complete weaning. Even though they may attempt to nurse after this time passes, rarely will this bring the mare back into any milk production or cause any problem. Some mares will have some secretion that can be "milked out" of their udders for months or even years after they have stopped normal milk production. Such a finding represents no problem or abnormality.

DRYING UP THE MARE

It should be remembered that it is the build-up of pressure that stops further milk production. The recommended procedure is to milk out a small amount of milk from the mare the first night only after the foal has been separated from her. This is to relieve some of the pressure, which will be uncomfortable for her. After that, no more milking is done. Further milking will only stimulate more milk production. The application of mild skin cream or hand lotion may be helpful to keep the skin from excessive drying from the normal congestion that will occur. Again, the use of aspirin (50 grains twice daily in a very little grain) will help greatly to minimize this udder congestion. No further treatment is usually necessary. Normally, most of the congestion, swelling, and discomfort will have subsided by the seventh day.

PART
III
Health Problems

CHAPTER

9

General Health Problems

The horse is commonly affected by abnormal conditions that influence its general health. The originator of the adage "healthy as a horse" was obviously not a horse owner. Horse owners can markedly reduce or minimize the effects of these conditions by knowing about them and utilizing good preventative medicine techniques. When we are conscientious, we can usually keep our horses in a good state of health and have many hours of pleasure and enjoyment. Most of the conditions that fall into the following categories are preventable: parasites, infectious diseases, noninfectious diseases, and injuries. *The most common universal affliction of horses the world over is internal parasites—worms.* All horses have some degree of infestation and should be routinely treated for it. Injuries are ranked second only to parasites as causes of abnormal conditions in the horse.

In general, horses are very accident-prone and owners need to take all steps necessary to eliminate possible sources of injuries. The most common cause of illness in the horse is an upper respiratory tract infection, a cold. Horses are very susceptible to these infections and the degree of seriousness varies depending on the cause and general resistance of the horse. There are vaccines that will protect against some of these infections.

In order for novice horse owners to be able to recognize common problems, the following is a description of a horse in good health.

SIGNS OF A HORSE IN GOOD HEALTH

General. A horse in good health should appear alert, with eyes clear and ears erect and active. It should stand with its feet square and firm on the ground. The alternate resting of the hind feet is normal, but the resting (pointing) of a front foot is an indication of a problem. A horse will almost always accept feed.

Coat. The hair coat should be sleek, shiny, and short during the summer months. During the winter, the coat is normally heavier and longer, but uniform in length, showing some sheen when groomed. It should not be greasy at its base, and the skin should not be scurfy.

Hooves. The walls of the hooves should be smooth and pliable. They should be rounded, not dished, misshapen, or splitting. The frogs should be well shaped, resilient, and touching the ground. There should be no thick, blackish, foul-smelling discharge (thrush) along the crevices of the frog. The digital pulse, which is felt just below the fetlock in the groove between the tendons and the pastern bone, is barely perceptible in the normal foot. A strong digital pulse indicates inflammation in the foot.

Temperature. The temperature of the horse has a normal range from 99 degrees in the morning to 101.5 degrees in the evening. Excessive exercise, especially on hot days, can elevate the temperature to 103 degrees or higher. A temperature of 103 degrees or more in a horse at rest usually indicates the presence of an infection.

Heart Rate. The normal heart rate of the horse should be between 28 and 52 beats per minute. Irregular beats are not uncommon and do not usually indicate a disease problem. A sustained rate over 80 indicates severe stress. The heart beats can be felt or heard through the chest wall behind the left elbow.

Respiratory Rate. The breathing, observed as flank or rib movements, should be noiseless and effortless. The normal respiratory rate is between 8 and 16 breaths per minute, but increases with exercise. A sustained rate of 100 or more is an indication of severe stress.

Defecation. A horse normally passes manure several times a day. It should be well formed but not excessively hard or mucous covered. The color will vary from a light tannish yellow to dark green, depending on the diet of the animal. Prolonged loose manure (over 3 days) or constipation should receive attention. Grunting during defecation is not uncommon.

Urination. Horses urinate a quart or more several times daily. The urine is normally thick and yellowish. Frequent, strained urination or only a small amount of urine being passed is abnormal.

WHEN TO CALL A VETERINARIAN

1. The horse completely refuses to eat.
2. The horse shows marked depression.

3. There is an excessive thick nasal discharge or any abnormal discharge.
4. The horse has frequent deep explosive coughing or a chronic cough.
5. The body temperature is over 103 degrees. The temperature can be taken with any human rectal thermometer.
6. There is evidence of colic, such as the animal getting up and down, rolling, kicking or biting at the flank, and sweating.
7. There is marked lameness (limping) or a mild lameness that persists over a week's time.
8. Frequent abnormal or unusual behavior is observed.
9. The treatment for severe wounds.
10. Routine care procedures such as parasite control, dental care, vaccinations, advice on nutrition, breeding problems, and general horse husbandry concerns.

CHAPTER

10

Parasites

INTERNAL PARASITES

There are over 150 different kinds of internal parasites of the horse now known. Most horses harbor some of these parasites in varying degrees of infestation. Though only a few of these parasites cause serious damage, they do frequently cause general debility, unthriftiness, and colic, not uncommonly resulting in sudden death. Most often the effects of parasites are brought about in a slow progressive manner and are not recognized as the cause of the damage. Indications of parasitism are general weakness, unthrifty appearance (often "pot bellied"), rough hair coat, poor growth, colic, and sometimes diarrhea (Figs. 72, 73, 74). Too frequently, only extreme symptoms are recognized by horse owners. It should be noted that not all horses are equally affected by parasites, but it is not uncommon to see fat, seemingly healthy horses heavily infested with internal parasites (Fig. 75).

The most serious damage is caused by the migration of these parasites through body tissues. It is during this migration that tissues are injured and pathways for bacterial invasions are created, which result in further tissue damage and occasionally in a generalized infection. Waste products of the migrating larvae often have toxic effects. Large populations of internal parasites within the intestinal tract can cause so much damage to the gut walls that proper absorption of nutrients is interfered with and poor utilization of feed results.

186

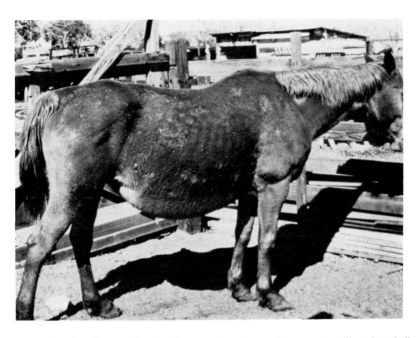

FIG. 72.   Mare heavily parasitized, with poor hair coat, poor flesh, and swelling along belly wall from anemia and low blood protein.

Strongyles

Strongyles, or blood worms, are the most consistently found parasite affecting horses throughout the world. It is very unlikely that any horse will live out its lifetime without having been a host to these worms. Over 90% of the horses that are autopsied at the University of California Pathology Department show blood vessel damage caused by this group of worms. Some forms are very destructive and are a common cause of fatal colics due to mechanical interference with blood supply to the intestine. The larvae of the large strongyles commonly damage the lining of the anterior mesenteric artery, which is the main source of blood to the intestines. The larvae cause a weakening of the vessel walls and a roughening of the inner lining. This results in an abnormal dilation of the vessel, which is called an aneurysm (Fig. 76). As blood passes by this roughened vessel lining, blood clots tend to develop. These clots are washed on down and block the smaller capillaries of the tissues of the intestines. Such blood clots are called emboli. The blocked blood supply to the tissue of the intestines causes gangrene of the intestinal walls, which then no longer function properly. The colic that results is called a thrombo-embolic colic and is usually fatal (Fig. 77). As a group, strongyles

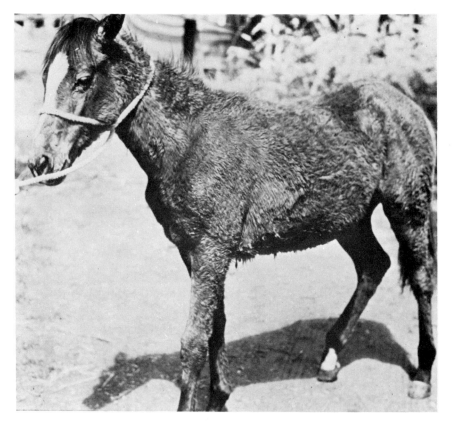

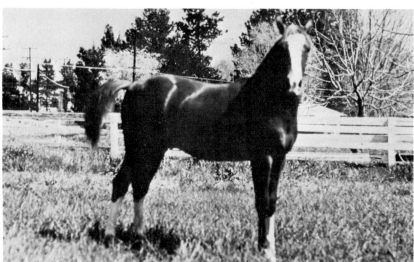

FIGS. 73 and 74.   Two six-month-old colts, one in good health and the other heavily parasitized.

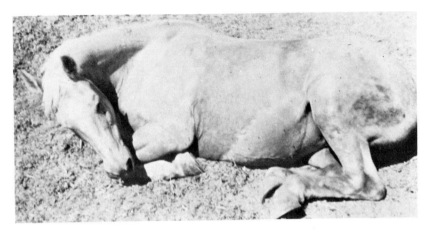

FIG. 75. A "fat" horse in good flesh in a fatal colic caused by blood worms.

are tissue feeders; they remove blood and can produce a toxin that causes blood cells to break down. Emaciation, anemia, soft bad-smelling feces, decrease in appetite, exhaustion, rough coat, stocking up of legs, colic, occasional diarrhea, and intermittent lameness are all symptoms brought about by these worms.

There are two main groups of blood worms: large and small. In general, the small strongyles (over 60 species) do not migrate through the body tissues, but remain within the confines of the gastrointestinal tract. The large strongyles are the most destructive because of their migrations through the body tissues. Strongyles are very prolific, and it is not uncommon to find as many as 1000 to 2000 eggs per gram of manure. Roughly, this means that such a horse will pass 20 to 30 million eggs a day in its manure. Depending on weather conditions, after 8 to 14 days, the eggs develop into infective larvae. Infective larvae are free living and crawl upon blades of grass, where they are picked up by grazing horses. These larvae are very resistant to drying and low temperatures and have been known to survive for several years in pastures or on the ground. Resting a pasture for only 2 months, however, significantly reduces the number of infective larvae. When ingested, the larvae remain in the intestines for about 2 weeks, after which they penetrate the gut wall. Some are picked up by the blood stream and carried to body organs, others travel through the body cavity to reach different structures such as the liver and pancreas (Fig. 78). Some larvae end up in the large blood vessels that supply the intestines and hind legs. This can happen to equines of any age and often causes death. By some unknown route, the larvae return to the caecum and colon, where they become adults and complete their life cycle. This process may take

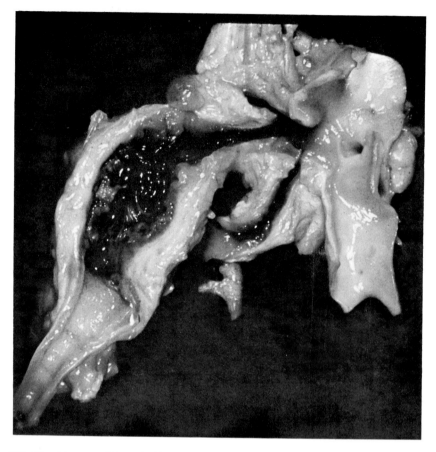

FIG. 76. "Aneurysm" in main blood vessel to intestines caused by blood worms. (Courtesy of Dr. J. H. Drudge, Lexington, KY.)

3 to 12 months, after which time eggs are again produced by those particular adults.

Control of strongyles is based on good sanitation and a routine worming schedule.

Ascarids

The large roundworms of horses are the most important parasites of young, growing horses (Fig. 79). This is one parasite that horses develop an immunity to, and it is very uncommon to find ascarids in horses over 5 years of age. Roundworms are particularly damaging because of the destruction that the migrating larvae inflict on the liver and lungs. Excretions of migrating larvae are often quite toxic to their host, and because of the large size and numbers of these worms, they occasionally cause partial or

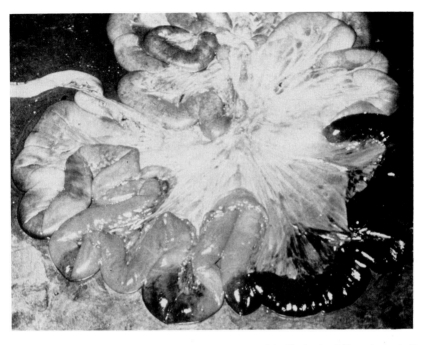

FIG. 77.   Loop of intestine damaged by blood worms caused death of animal (thrombo-embolic colic). (Courtesy of Dr. John Hughes, U.C. Davis, Calif.)

complete intestinal obstruction (Fig. 80). It is not known what the adult worms eat, but great tissue damage occurs during their presence. These, more than any other parasite, are the cause of pot-bellied, rough-coated, and stunted colts. The eggs are passed out in the manure and become infective in 10 to 15 days. They are very resistant and may survive up to 5 years on the ground, although they require some moisture. They will die in a few weeks if exposed to heat and dryness. Infective larvae are picked up in contaminated feed or water and are swallowed. Small larvae penetrate the gut wall and go to the liver, lungs, or other organs either by direct migration or by means of the blood stream. From the lungs they are coughed up and swallowed and they again return to the intestines where they develop into mature worms. The roundworms' migration through the tissues takes 21 to 30 days before they return to the gastrointestinal tract, and much damage occurs during this period. It is mainly because of this worm that we should conscientiously follow a vigorous worming program for all young horses, beginning at 8 weeks of age. This parasite commonly causes a dry, hacking cough in young horses.

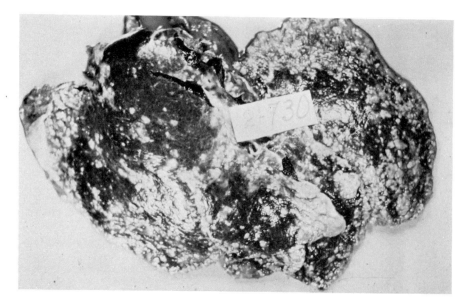

FIG. 78.   Damaged liver from migrating blood-worms. (Courtesy of Dr. J. H. Drudge, Lexington, KY.)

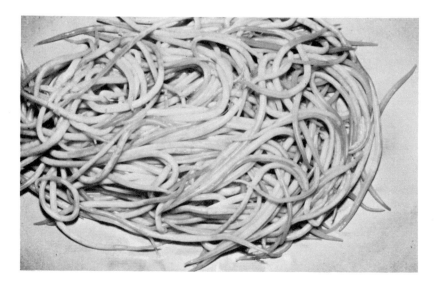

FIG. 79.   Ascarids from a colt. (Courtesy of Dr. John Hughes, U. C. Davis, CA.)

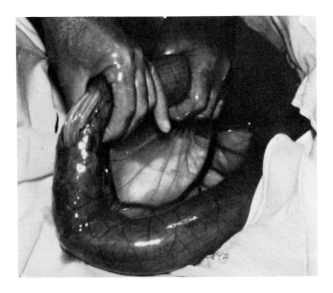

FIG. 80. Intestine blocked with ascarids being relieved surgically. (Courtesy of Dr. John Hughes, U.C. Davis, CA.)

Bots

These are flies that cause damage mostly in their larval forms, which attach themselves to the lining of the horse's stomach (Fig. 81). There they remain for 9 to 12 months, sucking blood and often interfering with normal digestion. When the larvae are passed out in the manure during the summer, they pupate in 2 to 4 days. The adult flies live only 5 days, not eating, and living solely to reproduce. Although they do not sting, their buzzing sound is quite disturbing to horses, as they deposit their eggs (500 to 1000) on the hairs of the legs, neck, and lips (Fig. 82). The eggs are stimulated to hatch by the warmth, moisture, and rubbing action of the horse's muzzle. After this stimulation, they hatch in 6 to 10 days and enter the mouth, where they migrate through the tissues of the cheeks, tongue, and pharynx (back part of the throat), taking approximately 3 to 4 weeks to reach the stomach. Frequently, the irritation of these parasites in the mouth promotes excessive salivation and causes horses to crib, and occasionally even makes them difficult to bit. There is an increase in fence-chewing during the months of October and November when the "bot" activity is at its height.

Adult flies don't enter buildings, won't cross over water, and do not fly at night. Massive numbers (which are not too uncommon) of the larvae, attached to the stomach walls, cause frequent

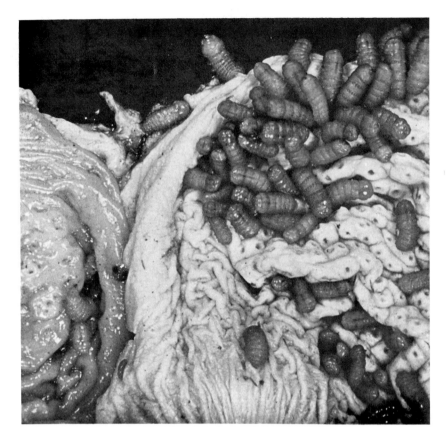

FIG. 81. Bot larvae attached to the wall of the stomach of a horse.

digestive upsets and colics, lowered vitality from poor digestion, occasional vomiting, and general debility resulting from toxemia.

Bots are best controlled by using a safety razor to remove eggs twice a week from the hairs where they have been deposited, and by worming twice a year.

Pinworms

These small white worms are very widespread and cause most of their damage by annoying horses while they lay their eggs (Fig. 83). This irritation results in tail-rubbing, restlessness, improper eating, loss of condition, and poor hair condition. The adult worms live in the large intestines where they mate, but the female goes to the rectum when it is time to lay eggs. She protrudes her tail out of the anus, and deposits cream-colored clusters of eggs on the adjacent skin. When she has finished her egg-laying duties, she dies. The eggs drop off onto the ground in 3 days, and hatch

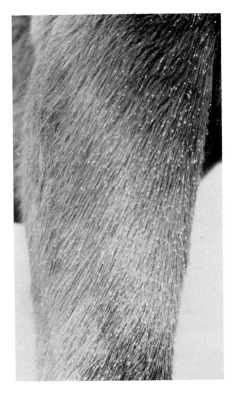

FIG. 82.   Bot eggs on the hairs of the legs. (Courtesy Dr. John Hughes, U.C. Davis, CA.)

in 5 days. The infective eggs are picked up by the horse via contaminated feed or water. Adult pinworms live on the vegetable matter of the intestinal contents, but the larvae feed on the gut lining. This parasite does no migrating through body tissues. Control is based on proper sanitation and a regular worming program.[11]

Stomach Worms (Habronema)

This is a worm of horses that is unique in that it requires the common house-fly as an intermediate host to complete its life cycle. The adult worms live in the stomach where they breed and lay eggs. The eggs are passed out in the manure. Maggots of the house-fly ingest these eggs and when the adult fly emerges, it carries in its body and proboscis the infective larvae of the stomach worm. Horses are usually reinfested when they accidentally swal-

---

[11]Pinworms of horses are not transmissible to children or vice versa.

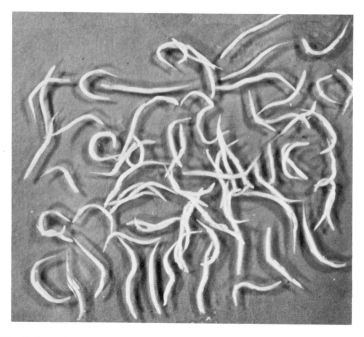

FIG. 83.   Mature pinworms. (Courtesy of Dr. J. H. Drudge, Lexington, KY.)

low such dead flies or when infective larvae are deposited on their lips by flies.

Though it is possible for these worms to occur in large numbers in the horse and cause stomach ulcers and poor general condition, this is not common. These parasites become most important to the individual horse whose wounds accidentally become infested with the larvae deposited there by a fly. These "displaced larvae" migrate through the tissues and make the wound very slow to heal. Such lesions are referred to as "summer sores," (Figs. 84 and 85).

Onchocerca

This is a parasite of horses whose importance has only recently been recognized. These hairlike worms live in the connective tissue of the neck. Adults produce larvae called microfilaria, which migrate through connective tissue and settle mostly on the underside, along the midline, from the chest to the inguinal area. Moist skin lesions frequently result, and it is through these raw areas that biting insects pick up the microfilaria and are capable of passing them on to other horses. A very irritating generalized

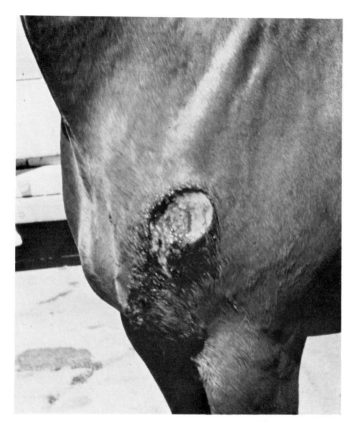

FIG. 84. "Summer sores" caused by the Habronema parasite deposited in the wounds by flies.

skin condition characterized by spots may result from this infestation.

Recently it has been found that this parasite frequently enters the eye during its migration. When the parasite dies within the eye, signs of periodic ophthalmia (moon blindness) develop. Studies indicate that this parasite may be the most common cause of this disease, but still other causes may be involved.

INTERNAL PARASITE CONTROL

Management

1. Provide sanitary feeding and watering facilities to prevent manure contamination.
2. Remove manure daily from stalls and at least weekly from paddocks.
3. Allow periodic 2-month rest periods of permanent pastures to reduce effectively infective parasitic larvae.

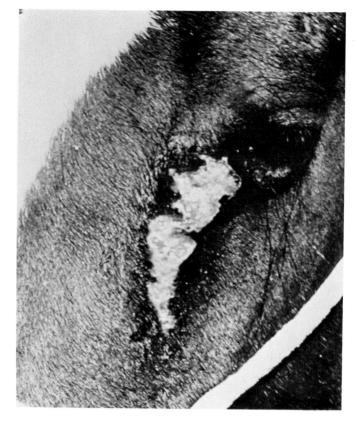

FIG. 85. "Summer sores" caused by the Habronema parasite deposited in the wounds by flies.

4. Avoid overcrowding to reduce parasite exposure.
5. *Never* spread fresh horse manure on pastures grazed by horses. Manure that has been composted for 2 weeks or longer is safe.
6. Worm all horses before putting them out on a new pasture.
7. Consistently follow an effective worming program.

Therapy

After reviewing the life cycles of the internal parasites of horses, it becomes apparent that, in the past due to internal larval migration, no single treatment was capable of eliminating all these parasites. This situation seems to have changed with the new systemic worm medicine, Ivermectin. Effective control is based on good management and routine worming. Since all worming medications are not equally effective, a veterinarian should be contacted for specific recommendations. It should be noted that garlic and tobacco have no value as antihelminthics.

WORMING SCHEDULE

It is advisable to worm all horses routinely twice a year for all four major groups of internal parasites (bots, strongyles, ascarids, pinworms). This is frequently done in the spring and fall, but there is no real need to adjust the timing with the first frost or a specific month. Spring worming often is coordinated with spring vaccinations. Because of the frequent rapid rebuildup of the populations of strongyles and ascarids, it is advisable to reworm for these parasites at 8- to 12-week intervals. Foals are first wormed at 8 weeks of age, but are not wormed specifically for bots until their first fall or winter. Pregnant mares, stallions in service, and working horses should be kept on this schedule with *proper medication*. Frequent worming of growing colts is especially important. Since all foals eat manure, it is advisable to worm pregnant mares late in pregnancy (30 to 40 days before they are due) to have her manure as free as possible of parasites. On farms where horses have been kept for years, monthly worming, especially for young animals, is a routine practice. Contact your veterinarian for a specific worming program.

EXTERNAL PARASITES

As with internal parasitism, external parasitism is a herd problem, rather than one of individual animals. Healthy, properly fed, well-managed animals have increased resistance to the invasion and establishment of parasites. Improper feeding and grazing, overstocking, unsanitary conditions, and poor attention to illnesses in their early stages all favor parasitism.

Lice

Lice of horses suck blood and can cause intense irritation, restlessness, loss of condition, rough hair coat, loss of hair, marked itching, and anemia. Common locations are the root of the tail, inside of the thighs, and along the neck and shoulders. It is thought that the lice claws and the nature of their saliva cause the acute discomfort of rubbing associated with louse infestation (Fig. 86). Horses affected by lice commonly have a "moth-eaten" appearance, frequently with many moist hair areas over the flanks where the horse has been biting itself. Many large areas of total hair loss are commonly seen.

Lice spend their entire life cycle on the host's body. Eggs, or nits, are attached to the hair near the skin, where they hatch in approximately 2 weeks. Two weeks after hatching, the young

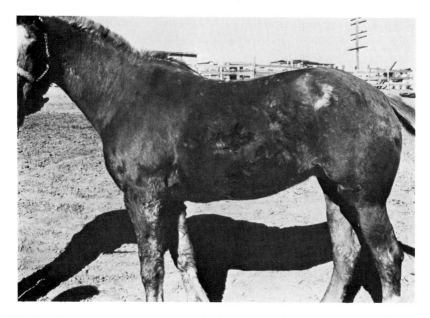

FIG. 86. Lice cause restlessness, intense itching, patchy hair loss, and sometimes diarrhea. Moist blotchy areas are frequently observed caused by the horse muzzling or biting at itself.

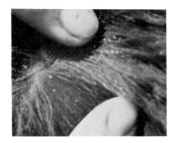

FIG. 87. Lice can be seen but are small and cream colored and often missed when one tries to find them.

females begin laying eggs again, after which they die. Lice do not live more than a few days off the host, and transmission is by direct contact and by contaminated tack.

Lice are quite specific to their desired host; that is, horse lice will not become established on cattle, chickens, or any other animals, and vice versa.

Horse lice are very small and, therefore, very difficult to see (Fig. 87). If horses are manifesting excessive rubbing and itching over many parts of their bodies, don't overlook the possibility of lice. Control is best accomplished by herd treatment (bathing) with an effective insecticide. Treatment should be repeated in 3 weeks in order to destroy lice hatching not affected by the first treatment. Lice powder can give temporary relief in cold weather.

Ticks

Ticks, in large numbers, are capable of causing severe anemia and even death; but even in small numbers, they can be important as a cause of irritation, restlessness, and spread of disease (Fig. 88). Ticks can be vectors of sleeping sickness, piroplasmosis, and equine infectious anemia (swamp fever). One species of tick is a frequent invader of the ears of horses and, because of the extreme irritation, often causes them to be difficult to bridle, droopy-eared, and head shy. Ticks, like mosquitoes, commonly cause skin bumps due to local allergic reactions to a toxin in their saliva.

Ticks, in general, are not very specific to any particular host. They seem to be just as satisfied dining on a deer, a horse, or a cow, and are most frequently found in low hills or bushy areas. It has been the author's experience that both ticks and lice are mostly a problem during the winter months. This is probably due to the lowered resistance horses experience from the stress caused by cold weather.

Adult females lay eggs (up to 18,000) on the ground and then die. The eggs develop into larvae that climb up on grass or shrubs where they latch on to a passing host. As each develops into a nymph, it sucks blood. Adults may breed either on or off the host, and ticks can frequently survive for long periods off the hosts— sometimes as long as 5 years (adults), or 6 to 12 months (immature forms).

Control measures are difficult. Removal of undergrowth in grazing areas helps, but the most useful and convenient control measure is the treatment of affected horses and other domestic animals

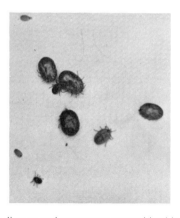

FIG. 88.   Ticks can carry disease and may cause severe blood loss.

that graze together with suitable insecticide baths or sprays. This not only reduces the effects of the ticks, but also cuts down on the number of potential egg-laying females and, if continued, permanently reduces the tick population. Good drainage reduces humidity upon which ticks depend. If they are prevalent in the stable area, it may be necessary to spray buildings. There is some clinical evidence that giving 2 tablespoons of Brewer's yeast daily in grain makes horses less palatable to ticks and lice.

Ear Ticks

The spinose ear tick has a larval form that crawls into the ears of horses, cattle, wild animals, sheep, and dogs and spends 1 to 7 months developing through the nymphal stage. They then drop out of the ears and crawl to fences, barns, feed bunkers, and trees to molt to adults, mate, and deposit new eggs. While in the ears of horses, they cause great discomfort and commonly cause the ears to be carried oddly to the side, often making the animals ear shy and difficult to bridle or halter. Contact a veterinarian for specific treatments. It should be noted that small-animals' ear mite medication is often effective.

Ringworm

Ringworm is caused by a fungus that is vegetative in nature, reproducing by asexual spores. Ringworm invades the hair and often the superficial layers of the skin, usually being introduced through a scratch that comes into contact with the spores. Lesions then develop as follows: at first, the hair is dry, scaly, and encrusted; then the infected hairs break off and the skin becomes scabby and sometimes raw and bleeding. At this time, the scab must be removed. Areas most commonly affected are the skin around the eyes, the muzzle, the neck, the saddle and saddle girth areas, and the root of the tail. Untreated areas often get large, and mild itching usually accompanies the disease.

Control measures involve treatment and isolation of the affected animal, and disinfection with a suitable fungicide of everything that has come in contact with the affected animal, such as grooming equipment, tack, and fences.

Warbles (Cattle Grubs)

This is mainly a parasite of cattle that sometimes accidentally affects horses. The harmful effect of these grubs on horses is the eruption of the larvae (grubs) on the animals' backs, frequently resulting in very tender, slow-healing sores that interfere with saddle horse usability.

Cattle grubs are the larvae of the heel fly, and the adults are

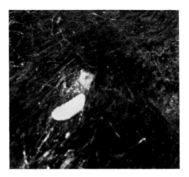

FIG. 89.   Warble being removed from the withers area of a horse.

rapid fliers that are very seldom seen. Their eggs, which are fastened to the hairs of the legs and body, hatch into small maggots, burrowing through the skin and migrating through the connective tissue of internal organs, body cavities, and the esophagus, where they remain until late winter, later migrating to the skin of the back. There, cysts are formed around each grub, and a breathing hole is established through the skin. In horses, these larvae frequently die, and never develop beyond the skin cyst stage. Because of this, they frequently must be surgically removed before healing will occur (Fig. 89). There are no specific preventative measures, although frequent application of fly repellents is helpful. The use of Ivermectin is proving effective.

Mosquitoes

The injury that mosquitoes inflict consists of severe annoyance, blood loss, local skin irritation (bumps), and occasionally, systemic generalized allergic reactions. They transmit sleeping sickness. Control locally is the same as for flies, but area control is a specialized procedure and should be in the hands of official agencies.

Flies

In general, flies can cause a great deal of annoyance and discomfort to the horse, to the point of causing them (especially the young) to run and occasionally hurt themselves. Some blood-sucking species have been linked with the spread of certain diseases such as anthrax, equine infectious anemia (swamp fever), sleeping sickness, and chronic abscesses (pigeon fever). When flies are present in large numbers, they can actually cause a significant blood loss.

Horseflies, deerflies, stable flies, horn flies, and face flies are the common species that affect horses and suck blood. The life cycle goes from adult to egg to larva (maggot) to pupa to adult. The time required for this cycle depends on the species and climatic conditions. Some cycles can be as short as 10 days. Flies survive the winter mainly in the larval form.

Horseflies and Deerflies

These usually attack horses as individual flies. Only rarely do they occur in large numbers, but as such, they can cause a significant blood loss. As many as 200 flies have been seen on a horse or deer and these would be capable of causing a blood loss of 100 ml or 3 ounces per day.

Stable Flies

While the larvae of horseflies are largely aquatic, stable fly larvae develop in moist fermenting vegetable matter and do not need manure. Their bite is more painful to livestock than most bloodsucking flies and can cause free flow of blood. Stable flies frequently occur in large numbers and livestock deaths due to massive infestation have been reported. Since stable flies visit their host infrequently and for short periods, they are best controlled by eliminating breeding areas and spraying their resting places (outsides of barns, fence posts, wooden fences, and tree trunks).

Horn Flies

The horn fly of cattle is a very common pest of horses and perhaps is the most annoying, due to the fact that they, unlike most other flies, spend most of their life on the host. They leave only to deposit their eggs in freshly dropped manure. Horn flies look very much like stable flies, but are only half the size.

The horn fly's life cycle, like that of the housefly, is among the shortest known for flies. Their eggs can hatch in less than 24 hours, the larval stage may be completed in 3 days, and the pupal period in 6 days, making a total of 10 days. Horn flies frequently occur in large numbers on the host—5000 to 10,000 have been reported on a single animal—and they feed twice a day.

Because of the bloodsucking habits of the horn fly and because it occurs in such large numbers over the entire United States, it probably is to blame for greater losses in livestock production than any other bloodsucking fly. Control in horses is basically dependent on disposal of manure and local applications of fly repellents on the animals.

Face Flies

The face fly is probably the most important insect pest to invade the North American continent during the past few years. This imported pest made its first known appearance in Nova Scotia in 1951. From 1951 to 1958 it became prevalent in areas of Canada. Since 1959 the face flies have spread over most of the United States, arriving in California in the late 1960s.

The face flies are appropriately named since the flies cluster or congregate in large numbers on the face and especially around the eyes of livestock. Cattle seem to be their preferred host, but horses are very commonly accepted as alternative hosts.

The flies have spongy mouthparts and feed on fluids excreted from the eyes and nose. The constant feeding and probing around the animal's eyes cause irritation and most likely transmit "pinkeye" of cattle and horses. Prior to 1970 the author never observed a contagious conjunctivitis ("pinkeye") of horses in many years of equine practice in northern California (Fig. 90). The condition became very common that summer and occurred in epizootic magnitudes. The condition is now becoming a common problem even in the early summer months.

The life cycle of the face fly is similar to that of the horn fly. The adult flies spend much of their time feeding or resting on the

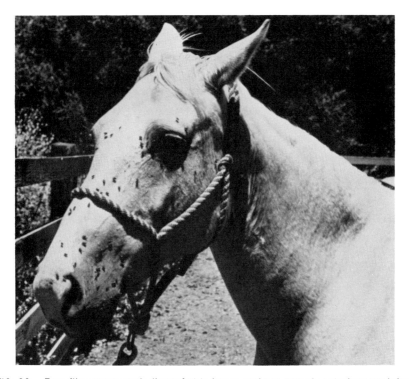

FIG. 90. Face flies cause much discomfort to horses and can spread contagious eye infections.

animal and the female flies deposit their eggs in fresh manure. After hatching, the larvae feed in the manure for several days before changing into the pupal stage. The pupae are bright orange in color and similar in size to the pupae of the common housefly. The period of time spent in the pupal stage may vary with the temperature. Warm, dry weather is most conducive to rapid development. The flies begin to feed soon after hatching and mating occurs shortly thereafter. When not resting or feeding on an animal, the flies may be found resting on posts, buildings, trees, or other such objects near the animals. During the winter months, they invade buildings or prefer to hibernate in warm attics.

Controlling face flies on animals is extremely difficult. Daily application of insecticide to the face of animals is effective and helpful, but most insecticides only last a few hours. Using face brow bands of cloth or leather with 6-inch strips hanging down from the band of cloth or leather over the face is often well tolerated by horses and is helpful to discourage the accumulation of flies around the eyes. The use of face screen masks can also be helpful. If used they should fit well and not be too close as to rub on the horse's eyes. Though many horses tolerate these well, many horses do not and soon rub them off. Oral feeding of an insecticide and salt mixture to cattle has proved effective in preventing development of the fly larvae in the manure, but this practice is only effective when the insecticide-salt mixture is widely used in an area because the flies can migrate long distances. Spraying resting places may further reduce their populations. The author opposes feeding an insecticide-salt mixture to horses where dosage is difficult to control.

Houseflies

Though the housefly is not a parasite of horses, it is an important pest of man and beast. Because the fly is attracted to animals' wastes for breeding, it is imperative that horsemen work closely with their neighbors and the Public Health Department to minimize it as a problem.

The housefly has a very short life cycle. Under warm climatic conditions, it is completed in as little as 10 days. A single female lays 5 to 6 batches of 100 to 150 eggs a little below the surface of organic deposits. They hatch in 8 to 24 hours. The larvae (maggots) develop in 4 to 8 days into the pupal stage. In 4 to 5 days, the adult fly emerges and it sexually matures in 2 to 12 days. Attractive materials for deposit of fly eggs are garbage, grass clippings, decomposing fruits and vegetables, animal and meat products, pet droppings, and animal manure.

General Fly Control Methods

Effective fly control depends upon two basic approaches: (1) sanitation to reduce fly breeding to a minimum and (2) chemical control to eliminate flies which do develop. Neither approach is satisfactory without the other, and both require continual vigilance.

SANITARY MEASURES

1. Remove manure daily from stables.
2. Remove manure weekly from paddocks and pastures.
3. Compost manure or spread thin to dry. If you spread in thin layers, do so outside of corral or pasture fences to reduce exposure of horses to parasite eggs. If you compost it, do it in a fly-tight box under polyethylene tarpaulins or a screen top, 2 to 4 weeks. Composting for 2 weeks kills all parasite eggs and makes it usable as fertilizer for horse pasture.
4. Compost also all grass clippings, leaves, dog droppings, and similar material or spread them thinly to dry.

   To make storage of manure convenient, it is suggested that a suitable manure box be placed near the stable or in each paddock. A box 6 × 12 × 4 feet made of 2 × 12 foot planks with a partition dividing it in half is satisfactory; the front should be made with removable planks to each half. It should be fitted with a screen top or kept covered with polyethylene tarpaulins. It is desirable to fence this box off from the immediate area of horse activity.

CHEMICAL CONTROL

Chemicals for fly control can be used as residual sprays, baits, space spray, and larvicides, as well as for direct applications on animals.

Residual Spray

Apply spray to those surfaces favored by flies for resting sites—inside and outside of the barn and corral fences—with residual spray. A simple hand trombone garden sprayer is satisfactory, applying to point of run off. Baiting the spray with sugar is mainly effective against the common housefly. Precautions: Since insecticides are toxic to humans and animals, follow manufacturers' instructions closely. Use gloves and wash well after applying insecticides. *Do not* spray hay, other feeds, or feed mangers, and *do not* contaminate the water supply. Remove animals from barn or corral before spraying and *do not* return them to the areas until the spray has dried.

Baits

Used alone, baits are not adequate to control a heavy fly population. Use weekly. Place bait in a safe place or container where children, animals, or pets cannot accidentally get the bait. A coarse screen box is satisfactory.

Space Spray

Used to rid and knock down flies in barns or where flies are numerous. No residual effect is achieved. Space sprays are best applied in fine mist or fog.

Larvicides

Used in emergency control of breeding in such areas as compost piles and garbage cans, action is relatively short.

Direct Applications on Animals

Spray or sponge on. Follow directions carefully as to proper dilution and application, since too highly concentrated solutions can cause toxic reactions and skin reactions. Water-diluted sprays cause less skin reaction than oil-base preparations.

Unfortunately, there is no fly repellent for the horse that seems to be effective for more than a few hours, but any repellent is worthwhile when it is locally applied for temporary relief.

Since new insecticide products are constantly becoming available, it is advisable to obtain specific recommendations from your veterinarian, farm advisor, or a pest control firm.

Note: The author has seen many horses have skin reactions to fly sprays that have an oil base that were used to "get ticks, too." Such preparations should be used very cautiously, if at all.

CHAPTER

11

Infectious Diseases

THE EQUINE RESPIRATORY COMPLEX

Respiratory diseases are the most common infectious disease problem in the horse (Fig. 91). They are second only to parasitism as a universal affliction of the equine species. The severity of the symptoms will vary from a mild nasal discharge to marked symptoms of a heavy nasal discharge, deep cough, lung congestion, and high fever, depending on the cause and complications.

Causes

We are able to clinically recognize three respiratory diseases caused by viruses and one caused by a specific bacterium. These diseases are known by the following names: (1) equine viral rhinopneumonitis, (2) equine viral arteritis, (3) equine influenza, and (4) strangles. Recently, new equine parainfluenza and rhinoviruses have been isolated but cannot be clinically distinguished from the other respiratory infections. Debilitated, excessively stressed animals are the most susceptible to these infections.

Prevention

All of the above respiratory infections are potentially contagious. Transmission is usually through direct contact with infected animals by rubbing noses, or indirectly from airborne secretions or contaminated water troughs. Affected animals should be isolated, if possible, for 2 to 3 weeks. Separate feed and water containers should be used. Avoid causing undue stress conditions by doing the following:

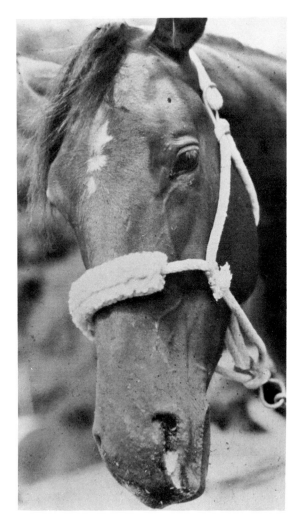

FIG. 91.   Respiratory diseases are the most common infectious disease problems in the horse.

1. Provide draft-free shelter during bad weather.
2. Avoid cold clammy barns.
3. Try to keep animals in good physical condition and in good flesh, and on a good parasite control program.
4. Do not allow exhausted, overheated, or debilitated animals to become chilled by turning them out hot; do not bathe animals on cold, windy days or ship them in a drafty, unprotected trailer.

It should be noted that a bran mash and the use of antibiotics before shipping increase the animal's resistance to respiratory infections.

Nursing and First-Aid

1. Allow complete rest during the period of illness and an additional 7 to 10 days to avoid serious relapses and complications.
2. Provide draft-free shelter.
3. Keep the animal warm with blankets, leg wraps, and heat lamps when the weather calls for it.
4. Dampen the hay and grain to keep down the dust, which irritates the already inflamed tissues of the nose and throat. Do not feed from overhead mangers.

Treatment

Proper treatment should be administered by a veterinarian. Antibiotics and cough medicines are frequently necessary. When an elevated temperature is present, aspirin (ten 5-grain tablets per 1000 pounds) dissolved in water and mixed in the grain is very helpful in reducing the inflammation and helps the horse's feeling of well-being.

Equine Rhinopneumonitis

This is a contagious viral disease that causes a mild upper respiratory infection, similar to the common cold in man, but may cause abortions in mares.

Cause

This disease is caused by a virus that is transmitted by direct contact and airborne respiratory secretions. Often, the initial source of the infection is not known. An outbreak may involve a large number of animals, but usually affects only 10 to 25% of the exposed horses.

Symptoms

Most affected animals develop a mild, watery discharge with an elevated temperature of 102 to 105 degrees. Coughing is not a predominant symptom. Recovery can be complete in 2 to 7 days if no complications occur. Thick nasal discharge, deep cough, and loss of appetite are signs of complications, and proper treatment is indicated.

This virus can cause abortion in mares and may cause "abortion storms" in a band of brood mares. This form of the disease is known as "equine virus abortion." Though equine rhinopneumonitis is common in the western states, abortions caused by the virus are relatively uncommon in the west.

Prevention

A good safe vaccine against this disease is available.

Equine Viral Arteritis

This is an acute contagious disease of horses that is characterized by a watery nasal discharge, inflamed eyelids, and frequently, swollen legs and ventral abdomen.

Cause

Equine viral arteritis is caused by a virus that is contagious and is capable of causing much tissue damage. Symptoms usually occur 2 to 6 days after exposure. Between 10 and 50% of the horses exposed to it develop the disease. The disease usually runs its course through a group of animals in 3 to 4 weeks.

Symptoms

Affected horses frequently become very ill with a fever between 103 and 106 degrees. The swellings of the eyelids and often the legs help distinguish this disease from other respiratory infections. A nasal discharge, which may become thick, is often accompanied by a deep cough. Symptoms usually subside shortly after the fever but may persist for 10 to 14 days. Pneumonia or a chronic cough may complicate the illness.

This disease has often been associated with the shipment of horses, and has been called "shipping fever." Debilitated, heavily parasitized, and malnourished animals are affected most severely. The virus can cause abortions in mares. Proper medical treatment is indicated.

Equine Influenza

This is an acute, highly contagious respiratory disease of horses that is characterized by a dry, hacking cough affecting almost all exposed, susceptible horses.

Cause

It is caused by a virus that appeared in the United States in 1963. It is now found in most countries. Most infections occur in the winter and the spring.

Symptoms

Affected animals develop a dry, hacking cough and often run a fever of 103 to 106 degrees for 2 to 5 days. A nasal discharge usually occurs after the onset of the coughing symptoms. Most affected animals show symptoms within 4 days after exposure. The very high percentage of affected horses in an outbreak is characteristic. While some horses only manifest mild effects, others may become very sick. Forced rest for 2 to 3 weeks following the illness is essential to prevent serious complications.

Prevention

A very effective vaccine is available for use against this disease. Its use is highly recommended, especially for those horses that are exposed to many other horses, such as race horses, show horses, and those kept at public stables. A veterinarian can provide specific recommendations.

Strangles

This is an acute contagious respiratory disease of horses that is characterized by a thick nasal discharge and the formation of a mandibular lymph gland abscess under the jaw (Figs. 92 and 93).

Cause

A specific bacterium, Streptococcus equi, causes strangles. The bacteria are found in the nasal discharge and the abscess pus. Young animals are the most susceptible and often have lifetime immunity after recovering from the disease. Most frequently, the source of infection in an outbreak is undetermined. Water troughs are ideal means of spreading the disease, especially when being used by a horse with a draining abscess.

Symptoms

Most affected animals first develop a watery, runny nose; the discharge then becomes thickish and then the development of the mandibular lymph gland abscess under the jaw is noted. A fever of 104 to 106 degrees accompanies the early symptoms. Although some horses become very sick, depressed, and "off feed," others show no obvious signs of illness, even though a mandibular abscess may develop and rupture by itself.

Symptoms usually occur 4 to 10 days after exposure. The course of the disease through a herd of horses is totally unpredictable. Sometimes only one or two horses develop the disease; at other times the disease may slowly work its way through a group, affecting almost every animal over a 3-month period. Affected animals usually recover in a 2-week period unless complications occur. The bacteria can settle in the lymph gland deep in the throat latch area and cause "strangling." Such animals should be seen by a veterinarian because the abscess must be carefully drained

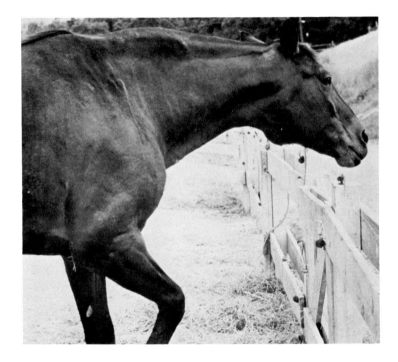

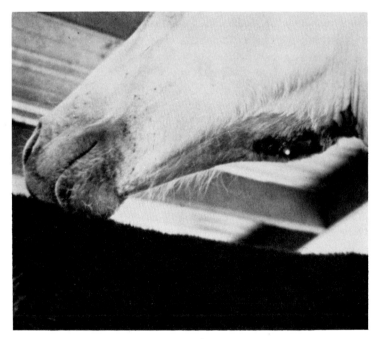

FIGS. 92 and 93.   An abscess under the jaw is characteristic of "strangles" infection.

without cutting vital blood vessels in the area. Internal abscesses occasionally develop and rupture, causing death.

Prevention

A vaccine is available for use against this disease. Because the disease occurs sporadically, the use of the vaccine is determined by the indications on the premises; certain breeding farms and public stables have histories of recurrent outbreaks of the disease. Contact your veterinarian for his specific recommendations.

Purpura Hemorrhagica

This is a disorder of the circulatory system that is characterized by generalized edema that most noticeably causes severe swelling of all four legs.

Cause

The disease is believed to be caused by an allergic reaction resulting from a streptococcal infection such as strangles. Viral respiratory infections are not known to be a cause, but may lower the horse's resistance to streptococcal infections. This is not a common disease problem.

Symptoms

The onset is usually observed 2 to 4 weeks after strangles or other respiratory disease that has resulted in a secondary bacterial infection. In early cases, most often the animal maintains a good appetite, stays alert, and has a normal temperature. As the swelling becomes extensive, the animal becomes very stiff and all four legs become very enlarged (Fig. 94). Often small purple spots (petechial hemorrhages) will be observed under the tongue or on the mucous membranes inside the lips. If it is untreated and the disease progresses, the head becomes swollen and breathing will be obstructed. The average mortality rate is 50%.

The course of the disease may vary from only 4 to 10 days in acute cases, but usually extends over a period of 2 to 4 weeks. Severe cases may require 2 to 3 months of convalescence.

Prevention

Since the disease is considered to be an allergic reaction of an individual, no specific preventative measures are known—except for the possible use of the strangles vaccine. Purpura hemorrhagica itself is not contagious.

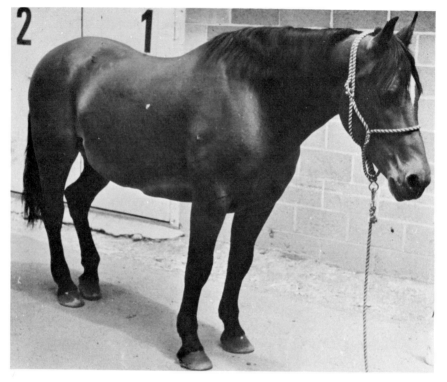

FIG. 94. Tissue swelling of legs and along abdomen are common symptoms of purpura hemorrhagica.

Nursing and First Aid

Proper treatment by a veterinarian is very important because the mortality rate is high. Prolonged use of antibiotics and cortisone drugs is indicated because the disease results from a deep-seated infection. The usual nursing methods for sick horses should be followed (see Chapter 13, Injuries and Treatment). The use of aspirin is helpful in further reducing tissue swelling.

Tetanus

This is an infectious disease of mammals caused by the toxins of the bacteria Clostridium tetani. It is characterized by increased reflex excitability of the motor nerve centers, resulting in spasmodic contractions of all voluntary muscles and usually death.

Cause

Clostridium tetani is a bacterium that is prevalent in soil and often in the digestive tracts of man and animals, especially horses. The spores are very resistant to all types of weather for a number of years. Although tetanus occurs most frequently in the warmer countries, it is considered to be worldwide in its distribution. Certain ranches and areas are heavily contaminated. The spores enter through wounds, although they must have an anaerobic (oxygen-free) environment in which to multiply before the toxins can be produced in sufficient quantity to cause symptoms. Frequently, however, horses suffering from this disease show no obvious wounds for entry of the spores. Even though deep punctures are the most ideal types of wounds for the bacteria, all wounds must be considered as possible sources for this disease. Young animals are the most susceptible, and the disease occurs most frequently during the wet spring and fall months when spores are washed to the surface of the ground.

Symptoms

The incubation period is 5 to 10 days but may be 60 days or longer. The first symptom in the horse is very characteristic and is diagnostic. It is the appearance of the *third eyelid protruding up* from the inner corner of both eyes, covering about one-third to one-half of the eyes (Fig. 95). Any excitement or sudden movements cause spasms of the muscles to the third eyelids and cause them to "flick" up and become very obvious as a covering over

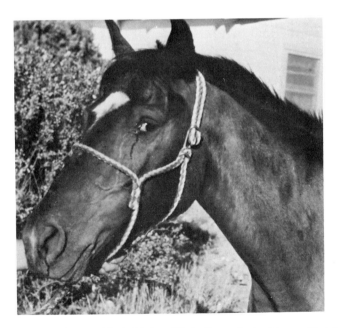

FIG. 95. The protruding up of both third eyelids is diagnostic for tetanus. Mortality rate is high. Prevention by vaccination should be routine for all horses.

the inner corner of the eyes. When the animal relaxes, the third eyelids temporarily become less obvious. As the disease progresses, the animal develops a general stiffness from overall muscle contractions caused by the tetanus toxin. Walking, turning, and backing are difficult. The animal may assume a "rocking horse" appearance. Spasms of the muscles of the head cause difficulty in chewing and may result in "lock jaw." The ears become erect and the tail becomes stiff. External noises can cause the animal to go into "tetanic" spasms. Death usually results from asphyxiation due to the persistent contraction of the respiratory muscles when the animal is down, sweating, and in a terminal convulsion.

Prevention

Besides vaccinations, good husbandry can be the most effective means of prevention. Pick up nails, tin cans, old farm tools, and other junk from areas where horses are kept. Good immunity to this disease can be developed from the use of *tetanus toxoid* vaccine. Because of the high susceptibility of horses and man to this disease, it is advisable for horses and horsemen to receive routine tetanus vaccinations. Consult a veterinarian and physician for their recommendations. *Tetanus antitoxin* should be used in the face of a wound in nonimmunized horses. This product provides immediate protection but only lasts approximately 2 weeks. The first toxoid vaccination and tetanus antitoxin may be given at the same time.

Nursing and First Aid

An affected animal should be placed in a quiet, darkened box stall. Place feed and water containers high enough so that the animal can use them without lowering its head. Avoid sudden movements or noises that might cause the animal to go into spasms. Proper medical treatment by your veterinarian is indicated. The use of massive doses of penicillin or broad-spectrum antibiotics, large doses of tetanus antitoxin, tranquilizers, and muscle relaxants has proven very effective in many cases. If symptoms come on slowly (over a 4- to 7-day period), the chances are better for the horse's survival. The average mortality rate is 80% in untreated cases.

Sleeping Sickness (equine encephalitis)

This is an acute viral disease of horses that may also affect man, other mammals, birds, and reptiles. It is characterized by central nervous system disturbances.

Cause

There are presently five known viruses that can cause encephalitis in horses throughout the world. The diseases are called *Eastern, Western, Venezuelan, Japanese,* and *St. Louis* encephalitis.

Eastern and Western Encephalitis

The Eastern and Western viruses are the principal causes of the disease in the United States. The Venezuelan virus has been identified in Texas. The Japanese encephalitis is an Asian disease. The St. Louis virus occurs throughout the United States but appears to cause no symptoms.

Transmission of the disease is mainly through mosquitoes, in which the virus is capable of multiplying. It persists in the salivary glands. Affected birds, which may show no symptoms, may act as reservoirs in nature. Susceptible birds include pheasants, chickens, ducks, turkeys, quail, blackbirds, and many others. Horses affected with the Western virus do not develop a stage where the virus is found in the blood stream, therefore are considered dead-end hosts, and cannot pass the disease on from biting mosquitoes. Horses with the Eastern virus may have a short period of being a source of infection when the virus is circulating in the blood stream (viremia), but this occurs before the horse shows any symptoms. Unlike the Eastern or Western viruses, the Venezuelan virus produces a long viremic stage and can be spread by direct contact.

Symptoms. Affected animals will initially develop a fever from 103 to 107 degrees. There is a reduced appetite accompanied by signs of difficulty in chewing and swallowing. The animal may submerge his whole head when attempting to drink. Frequent yawning, grinding of the teeth, circling, and stumbling are common symptoms (Figs. 96 and 97). Impaired vision, depression, and incoordination are further signs of brain involvement. Inability to rise and paralysis are terminal signs. Mortality rate is between 20 and 90%, depending on the particular virus causing the outbreak. The virus localizes in the brain and destroys the nerve cells.

Prevention. Annual vaccinations in the spring are recommended in areas where the disease is prevalent. Mosquito control is helpful.

Nursing and First Aid. Good nursing, aspirin, and supportive treatment by a veterinarian often help in the recovery of mild cases, but recovered animals frequently exhibit permanent signs of brain damage.

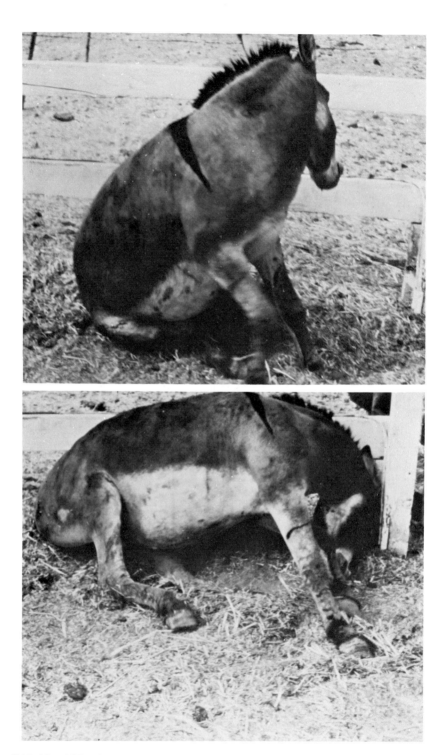

FIGS. 96 and 97.   Sleeping sickness is characterized by incoordination, circling, and pushing up against solid objects.

Venezuelan Equine Encephalomyelitis

This was first reported as a recognizable disease of horses in the U.S. in Texas on July 1, 1971. It resulted in 1500 deaths within 6 weeks. Prior to 1970, the disease had mostly restricted itself to South and Central America but the disease did make its way up into Mexico in 1970, killing several thousand horses that year. The 1971 outbreak in Texas caused the government to instigate mandatory vaccination programs in many states to protect the horses of the United States.

The virus primarily affects horses and humans. Though the mortality rate in horses may be up to 90% or more, the disease generally is mild in humans, causing signs resembling influenza— mild general discomfort, fever, and sore muscles and joints. The virus is capable of progressing into encephalitis and is more common in children and aged persons.

Transmission is mainly through mosquitoes. Rodents and other small mammals may be reservoirs for the virus. Birds are not as important as a source of this sleeping sickness virus as they are for the Eastern and Western varieties.

Symptoms. Affected horses may show signs of the disease within 1 or 2 days of exposure. The virus may last 1 to 6 days in the blood stream of a diseased horse, during which time it is a source from which the virus can be spread to other animals. Some horses may become infected and develop an immunity without showing clinical signs. Early signs are fever, depression, loss of appetite, and occasionally, abdominal distress and diarrhea. As the disease progresses, the "twitching" reflex of the skin is lost, the lips droop, and the pupils may contract. The animal may appear blind, have convulsions, and hang its head or press it against a wall, post, or other immovable object. Stumbling, circling, and "sleepwalking" are late signs. Eventually, the horse sinks to the ground and is unable to get up. Death often results 3 days after the first symptoms.

Prevention. Mosquito control and vaccinations are methods being used. The vaccines for the Eastern and Western encephalitis viruses does not confer immunity against the Venezuelan equine encephalitis virus. Consult a local veterinarian for specific advice.

Chronic Abscesses

This is a bacterial disease of horses that is characterized by large abscesses in the chest, lower abdominal wall, and/or the sheath or mammary area. This disease has in some areas been referred to as "pigeon fever." This terminology most likely started because of the enlarged chest area from developing abscesses, which appears to resemble the breast of a pigeon. The disease has no known connection to pigeons and this terminology should be discouraged.

Cause

The specific causative bacterium is Corynebacterium pseudo-tuberculosis, though in some areas a staphylococcus bacterium has been incriminated. This Corynebacterium has long been known to cause abscesses in sheep in the western hemisphere, but only in the last two decades has it become a common cause of abscesses in horses in the Western United States. The exact means of spreading of the infection is not clearly understood, but flies are believed to be the main vectors. The disease is most prevalent in the late summer and fall, corresponding to the peak fly season. The area on the lower abdominal wall, which frequently becomes raw from fly irritation, is thought to be a possible means of entry for the bacteria.

Symptoms

Most often a large single swelling (abscess) will develop on either side of the chest muscles (Fig. 98). At times, this will develop in a matter of only a few days, while at other times it may take weeks to build up, become soft, and be ready to break. The abscess material is typically a thick yellowish material. The disease may take the form of multiple small abscesses in the chest area or single abscesses along the lower abdominal wall, in the sheath or mammary area, or less frequently, on the face or along the vulva or hind legs (Figs. 99 and 100). Occasionally, internal abscesses develop and result in the death of the animal. The course of the disease in a single animal or a group of horses is totally unpredictable. Most often an individual animal will be affected from 4 to 6 weeks, but this time period is widely variable.

Prevention

No commercial vaccine is presently available to be used against this disease. Frequent use of fly repellents may be helpful. It is also helpful to keep any moist area along the ventral abdominal wall sprayed with yellow topazone to keep it dry and not attractive to flies. The isolation of an affected animal may be of value but is not a routinely recommended procedure (horses are not considered directly contagious).

Nursing and First Aid

The sooner the abscesses build up and drain, the shorter is the recovery period. Early use of antibiotics may be helpful, but some

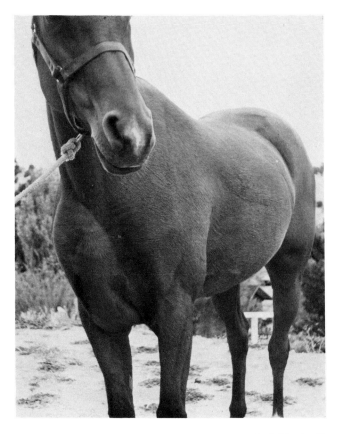

FIG. 98. Chronic abscesses are a common late-summer problem in California. Chest abscess is seen here.

veterinarians feel their early use may prolong the course of the disease. The treatment procedure should be at the discretion of your veterinarian. The author believes that antibiotics may help prevent the infection from spreading deeper into the body and thus are indicated. Running hot (120 degrees) water on the area is helpful. The application of hot towels soaked in warm Epsom salts solution (2 cupfuls to a gallon of water) to the area for a 15- to 20-minute period twice daily is helpful. A flaxseed poultice may be used and is made by boiling 2 cupfuls of flaxseed in 3 cups of water. This is boiled to a doughlike consistency. While this is cooling down, add 1 teaspoon of sodium bicarbonate and mix thoroughly. This material is then spread between two dishtowels or pieces of aluminum foil and held in place over the abscess. When the abscess ruptures, the cavity may be flushed with a suitable disinfectant. The use of petroleum jelly below the drain-

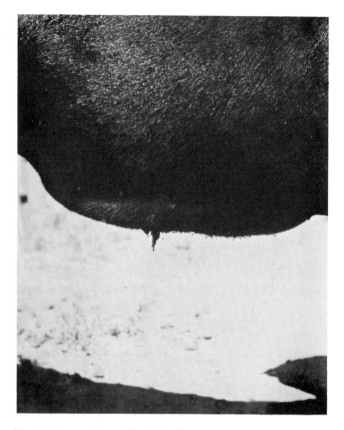

FIG. 99. Chronic abscess along abdominal wall.

ing abscess helps protect the skin from irritation. The edges of the wound should be treated with a fly repellent.

Equine Infectious Anemia (Swamp Fever)

This is a disease caused by a virus that is characterized by intermittent fever, depression, progressive weakness, loss of weight, leg edema, and anemia (Fig. 101). It is found in most countries of the world.

Cause

The virus is most often introduced in the horse by mosquitoes and other bloodsucking insects. The use of contaminated hypodermic needles or surgical instruments can be a cause. The disease usually spreads slowly and individual cases are observed sporadically. Once an animal becomes infected, it usually becomes a carrier of the virus for the remainder of its life. The virus has been found in the blood, nasal secretions, urine, milk, and semen of

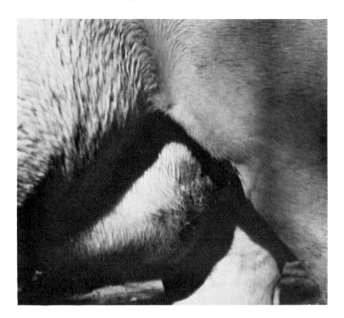

FIG. 100.   Chronic abscess in sheath area.

infected animals. Because of this carrier problem, known infected animals are best destroyed. The disease is most prevalent in areas where mosquitoes thrive. The disease is relatively uncommon in California.

Symptoms

It usually takes 1 to 3 weeks from the introduction of the virus into the horse before symptoms occur. The disease may be very mild or may be very acute, causing death in less than 7 days. Usually the animal will develop edema or swelling in all four legs. There often is an undulating rise in temperature. The animal loses its appetite and loses weight rapidly. Anemia results in pale gums and a generalized weakness. Many cases have a prolonged period of illness lasting over several weeks. The average mortality rate varies from 30 to 70%. There is a blood test that has been developed to diagnose the disease and many countries are now testing all horses before they are allowed inside their borders.

Prevention

None is known. Only symptomatic treatment and good nursing procedures are used in the case of the sick animals. There is a laboratory test called the "Coggins Test" that can identify animals that are affected with the disease or that are carriers. Many states now require this test before they allow outside horses to enter

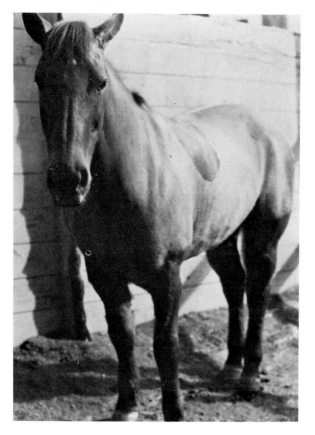

FIG. 101. Horses with equine infectious anemia (EIA) often look like "purpura" cases but a blood test is diagnostic.

their borders. Because no set procedures have been established to handle positive reactors, the use of this test to control the disease is very controversial within the veterinary profession. Positive animals are best protected from biting insects as much as possible to prevent possible spread to other animals.

12

Noninfectious Diseases

INTERNAL DISORDERS

Colic

Colic is a general term used to indicate pain in the abdominal cavity. There are many causes of colic, which is the major cause of death in horses. All cases of colic should be considered serious.

Clinically, colics fall into two main types: (a) excessive intestinal activity (hyperperistalsis), which is characterized by many loud sounds heard by placing the ear next to the horse's abdomen and (b) reduced intestinal activity (hypoperistalsis or aperistalsis), which is characterized by few or no intestinal sounds heard through the abdominal wall. The first type has been classically described as *spasmodic colic*. The second type has been called *flatulent* or *gas colic* because gas most often builds up within the intestinal tract when the intestinal tract stops functioning normally. This occurs in the case of an impaction. "Bloating" or abdominal distension is most often an advanced symptom of an impaction, usually of 24 hours' duration or longer.

The causes of both forms are similar but their degree of seriousness is markedly different.

Causes

1. Parasites may cause irritation to the intestinal tract, causing spasms. They may block the blood supply to the intestines and cause death.
2. Moldy or spoiled feeds are always a potential cause of acute

intestinal irritation and serious colic. They may be poisonous to the horse and usually cause acute intestinal spasms.

3. Sudden changes in feed, ingestion of foreign bodies, over-eating of grain, eating grain when exhausted, drinking too much water when hot, and feeding on sandy ground are common causes of gas colic.

4. Horses' teeth grow throughout their lives and usually need to have the sharp points filed (floated) once a year to assure proper chewing of feed to prevent impactions and to improve digestion. Teeth with sharp edges or long points cause pain to the horse while chewing, and this results in feed not being well chewed before being swallowed. This coarsely chewed hay predisposes the animal to intestinal obstruction. Aged horses with this problem and a less resilient and active digestive tract (often with inadequate exercise) are more prone to intestinal obstructions from these causes. Faulty teeth and the collection of sand in the intestinal tract are the most common causes of recurrent colics. Damaged intestines from worms can also be a common cause of recurrent colic.

Symptoms

Uneasiness, pawing, looking at flanks, kicking at the abdomen, sweating, getting up and down, rolling, resting in odd positions, such as on haunches or back, are common symptoms (Figs. 102 and 103). Severely congested inner eyelids (a bright red to a brick brown) accompanied by an elevated heart rate of 80 to 100 beats per minute or more, along with the lack of normal abdominal sounds, are signs of a poor prognosis and frequently a terminal outcome.

Prevention

Become familiar with the common causes of colic and take measures to avoid those conditions. Never offer a feed that might possibly be defective. "If in doubt, throw it out." It might turn out to be the most expensive feed you ever fed.

Nursing and First Aid

If the animal is passing manure and/or much intestinal rumbling can be heard through the abdominal wall, it most likely is having *spasmodic colic*. The symptoms may be acute, but the prognosis is usually good unless there is acute diarrhea and there are signs of shock. The animal should be kept quiet, if possible, and should be prevented from hurting itself. Quiet walking for 10 to 15 minutes of every hour may help distract the animal from the pain, but it should not be mounted and forced to exercise; this causes

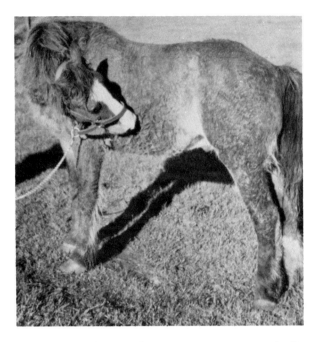

FIG. 102. Looking at and kicking at the flank are common symptoms of colic, as are getting up and down, pawing, and rolling.

undue stress, and may hasten a fatal outcome. If the horse wants to lie down in between the periods of quiet, forced walking, this is perfectly permissible; it might be able to rest or find a more comfortable position. There is very little danger of any rolling causing a twisted intestine. The horse might actually be able to relieve a gas accumulation. There should be no hard and fast rule not to allow a horse with colic to get down and roll if the animal is not frantic and not hurting himself. The offering of a bran mash[12] with aspirin in early cases of spasmodic colic often gets the animal over the problem with an uneventful recovery. If the animal is not definitely improving within 30 minutes after the offering of the bran mash, professional help should be sought.

If the animal refuses the bran mash, the aspirin will still be helpful. Crush up the 10 aspirins, mix them with a small amount of honey, and gob the mixture into the corner of the horse's mouth.

---

[12]Bran Mash: Put half of a 16-ounce box of 100% or 40% All Bran—Nabisco or Kellogg's— cereal or a 1-pound coffee can of wheat bran in a bucket. To this add very hot water to make it sloppy wet. Then add enough of the usual grain feed—oats or mixed grain— until the mixture is no longer sloppy wet but just warm and dampish. To this add 2 tablespoons of baking soda and 10 aspirins (dissolved).

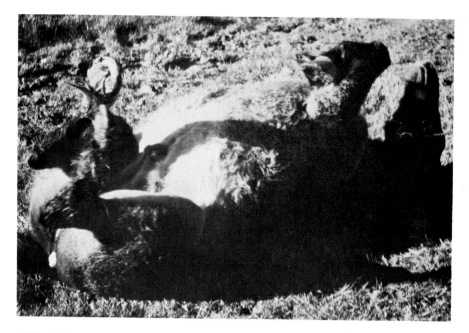

FIG. 103.   Horse rolling because of pain from a severe terminal colic caused by parasites.

If the animal is not passing manure and no abdominal sounds are heard, with or without signs of bloating, and the symptoms of pain are acute, professional help should be obtained as soon as possible. These are symptoms of a nonfunctional intestinal tract, which is always serious. Quiet walking 15 minutes every hour is indicated as a first-aid measure. Excessive walking can cause additional stress to the animal, but this exercise is often helpful to stimulate normal activity of the digestive tract. The use of intravenous fluids, analgesics (to control pain), steroids, and antibiotics by the attending veterinarian can greatly help to give physiological support to the animal to combat the stress of the situation. These animals are usually in great distress and no attempt should be made "to ride the colic out of them." Do not put irritating objects into the rectum.

If veterinary care is not available within a relatively short period (4 to 8 hours), the careful administration of milk of magnesia (16 ounces) with a turkey-basting syringe is indicated. This can be done by holding the horse's head slightly elevated (while the horse is standing). The contents of the basting syringe is slowly expressed into the mouth at the corner of the lips. Allow the horse to make voluntary swallows. *Do not* attempt to give such medication while the horse is lying down. It should be noted that the giving of mineral oil by forcing it into the mouth is very dangerous because it can get into the lungs easily. Unfortunately, too many cases of colic are overtreated, and this overtreatment is often the direct cause of death. A mild, shallow, and soapy (1 to 2 gallons) warm-water enema may be helpful for low impactions. Rectal tissues are easily damaged; care must always be the rule when this area is examined or receives medication.

Early detection and treatment of a severe impaction or other serious intestinal problem by your veterinarian can greatly improve the horse's chances of survival. Recently developed diagnostic techniques can help a veterinarian recognize which colic cases need surgery while the animal is still a good surgical risk. Successful equine abdominal surgery is now commonplace.

Laminitis

Laminitis (founder) is an inflammation of the sensitive laminae of the foot. It usually affects both front feet, but all four feet may be affected. It is characterized by stiffness and a "walking on eggs" gait.

Causes

Congestion within the hoof, which cannot swell from the inflammation, causes great pressure on the nerves and results in severe pain. The following are conditions that are known to be causes:

1. Hooves being trimmed too closely. Animals that are easily affected should have their hooves left a little long.
2. Overeating of grain. It usually takes 25 pounds or more to bring about symptoms.
3. Ingestion of unlimited amounts of cold water by an overheated animal.
4. Excessive use on hard ground or road surfaces causes "road founder."
5. Hard work by an unconditioned animal.
6. Toxemia from post-foaling retained afterbirth or uterine inflammation.
7. Lush green grass given to hypothyroid horses. These animals typically have large, heavy crests. Normal horses do not seem to "grass founder."

Symptoms

Tenderness on both front feet or all four is noted. Acute lameness is present and the animal will have a "walking on eggs" appearance (Fig. 104). The hind legs will often be placed well forward under the body to take as much weight as possible off the front legs. The affected feet will be warm (it is often very difficult to detect abnormal heat in the hooves by feeling), and there will be a strong digital pulse.

Nursing and First Aid

Professional treatment is indicated and highly recommended to help avoid the chronic form of this disease which may take months for recovery. Initially, a bran mash is beneficial. The giving of Dristan (8 to 10 tablets per 1000 pound horse) or other suitable antihistamine or aspirin twice daily in a minimal amount of grain is helpful, or can be medication prescribed by a veterinarian. Soak the feet in a mud bath, stream, or soaked burlap sacks for 2 to 6 hours daily for the first 2-week period or longer, as needed.

In chronic cases, the grooving of the hooves by a veterinarian is often helpful in relieving pressure and hastening recovery (Fig. 105). A "dropped sole" is the name given to the condition of the third phalanx separating from the inner hoof attachment and pressing down on the sole, and may be a complication of this disease (Fig. 106). New treatments have been helpful in some such cases. Bar shoes with pads or stainless steel plates often give relief to the animal that is making a slow recovery. Acupuncture may be helpful.

Lumbar Myositis

Lumbar myositis (sore back) is a muscular disorder of horses that is characterized by tender muscles over the loin area. "Tying

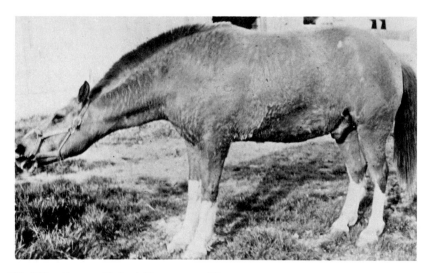

FIG. 104. Horses with laminitis are very stiff and usually are reluctant to move any more than necessary.

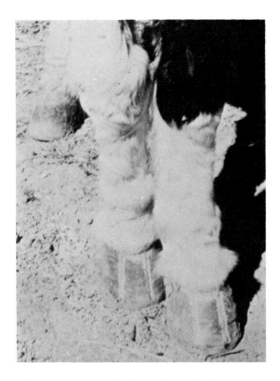

FIG. 105. Grooving the hooves in an effective method of treating chronic cases of laminitis.

up" is believed by many to be a less severe form of azoturia (Monday-morning sickness), both of which result in sore backs.

Cause

The exact etiology of the disease is not clearly understood, but much evidence indicates that an imbalance in the calcium-phosphorus ration in the diet may be a primary factor, though some animals develop symptoms when receiving a balanced ration. Too little calcium with an excess of phosphorus in the diet will bring on symptoms. A diet of poor-quality grain or grass hay, or poor-quality pasture, while also feeding a large quantity of oats, barley, bran, or combinations of them, is a typical imbalanced ration. An inflammation to the bursa (trochanteric bursitis) and related fascia (connective tissue) over the femurs (heavy bones of the hindquarters) has been recognized to be a cause of secondary sore back. Horses trying to compensate for inflammation in this area develop sore back muscles. Steroids or sclorosing agents have proven useful for treating this condition. The intramuscular injection of a female hormone may help by relaxing involved ligaments.

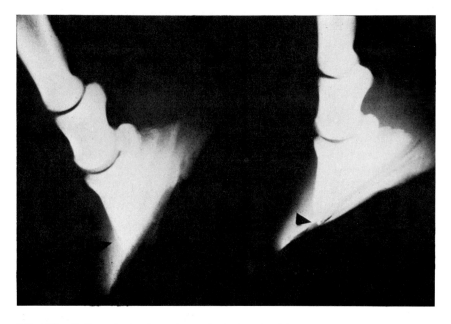

FIG. 106.   Radiograph showing a dropped sole from laminitis. If this occurs, there is little hope of having the animal normal again.

Symptoms

If firm pressure is applied with the fingers over the back muscles, the animal shows evidence of discomfort and may almost drop to the ground if it is severely affected. A normal horse should be able to take extreme pressure over the back and show no discomfort. Many affected animals are reluctant to work and may drag the toes of the hind hooves. In an animal showing evidence of "tying up," the back muscles become very rigid, stiffness of the gait develops, and sweating may occur. With azoturia, the animal is unable to move forward and the loin muscles are extremely hard. Forced exercise worsens the condition. A black-coffee-colored urine may be noted. Azoturia usually occurs the day after a day or rest while the horse is on a full, heavy grain ration.

Nursing and First Aid

In mild cases, a 7- to 14-day rest period along with a reduced grain ration and a balanced diet is all that is needed. Mild cases of "tying up" may be quietly walked. In more advanced cases, the animal should be rubbed dry, blanketed, stabled, and allowed to rest. Medical treatment is indicated when symptoms are pronounced. Selenium and vitamin E therapy has been effective in the treatment and for the prevention of this disease problem. The addition of 2 tablespoons of Brewer's yeast (vitamin-B complex help in muscle metabolism) in the grain once daily with or without 4 tablespoons of calcium lactate or powdered milk is helpful. The feeding of a good-quality hay (alfalfa is an excellent natural source of calcium) with a balanced grain ration is important.

Yellow Star Thistle Poisoning

Yellow star thistle poisoning is a disease caused by eating the Yellow Star Thistle plant (Centaurea solstitalis) and is characterized by the animal being unable to pick up, chew, or swallow feed. The odd chewing movements that occur account for the disease being referred to as the "chewing disease" (Fig. 107).

Cause

The Yellow Star Thistle plant, especially common in northern California, is the cause of the disease. It is an annual weed that is found along roadsides and in pastures. A toxic principle in the plant only affects horses and damages the particular part of the brain that controls chewing and swallowing. It usually requires at least 3 weeks of exposure and eating of the plant before symptoms occur. Some animals actually develop a taste for the plant and seek it out. Providing good feed for exposed animals is definitely advisable, but may not prevent the animals from eating the plant. The plant is potentially dangerous in all stages of

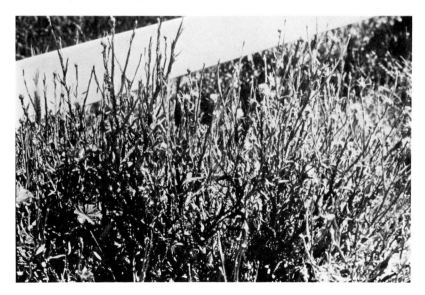

FIG. 107. Yellow star thistle poisoning is mostly a problem in northern California.

growth, even in hay, but most cases occur in the summer and fall.

Symptoms

An affected animal appears to have difficulty in picking up feed, and when feed is in the mouth, he is unable to chew or swallow it. Some of the feed often falls back out of the mouth. The chewing movements frequently appear involuntary and the mouth is commonly held open (Fig. 108).

Prevention

Avoid pastures and hay infested with Yellow Star Thistle if possible. The plant can be sprayed with 2-4-D or other weed killer in its growing period. Since it is an annual plant, spraying is a help in controlling it, as is physical removal by weeding or plowing under before it goes to seed.

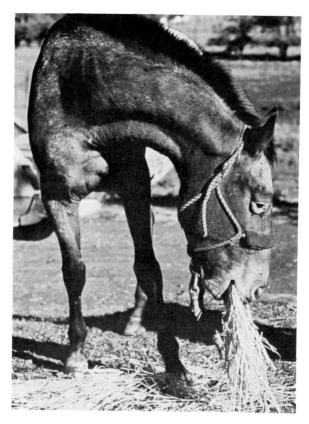

FIG. 108.   Affected horses lose control of chewing because of brain damage and would starve to death if they were not euthanized.

Nursing and First Aid

Yellow Star Thistle causes permanent brain damage and there is no treatment. The animal eventually dies of starvation or thirst if it is not euthanized.

Heatstroke

Heatstroke (overheating) is a disease that results from a disturbance of the heat-regulating mechanism of the body. It is characterized by signs of weakness, tremors, and elevated body temperature.

Cause

Prolonged hard or fast work during hot weather. Young, poorly conditioned animals and those with long-hair coats are most susceptible.

Prevention

Have animal well conditioned for hard rides. Clip heavy coats, water frequently (but in limited amounts when animal is hot), and avoid overtaxing the animal.

Symptoms

Initially, rapid breathing, weakness, stumbling, and sometimes refusal to continue working. In all cases, *sweating stops* and the skin becomes dry. This is an important early sign that heatstroke is about to occur. An *elevated temperature* of 106 to 110 degrees is diagnostic. The animal may show evidence of delirium and convulsions. Death may occur within 2 hours if the animal is not cooled off and does not receive proper medical treatment in advanced cases.

Nursing and First Aid

The aim is to reduce the high body temperature. The body should be sprayed with cold water. Ice packs to the head are indicated if the animal shows any sign of incoordination. After the body-temperature is lowered, the animal should be rubbed dry to prevent chilling. Medical treatment for shock is indicated for serious cases.

Exhaustion

Exhaustion is the result of overexertion and is characterized by inappetence, thirst, cold sweating, and weakness.

Cause

Overwork or use, especially when not well conditioned.

Symptoms

Weakness, refusal to eat, especially grain, and thirst. The body is usually clammy and *sweating is often patchy.* The body temperature may be normal or slightly elevated. The animal may desire to lie down. "Thumps" (spasms of the diaphragm) may occur and will cause spasmodic jerking in the flanks.

Nursing and First Aid

Attempt to make the animal comfortable. Cover the body with a blanket to prevent chilling. Do not force it to exercise if it wants to lie down. Hand rub its legs. Allow frequent limited quantities of water. When it is well rested, it will resume eating. Never feed grain to an exhausted animal. Hay is always safe. Many animals refuse to eat for some time after a hard ride; this is not serious unless other signs of fatigue are present. If "thumps" are observed, complete rest is indicated along with plenty of fresh air, but without drafts. The use of an antispasmodic injection by a veterinarian may be indicated for severe cases or for those making a slow recovery.

COMMON SKIN CONDITIONS

Horses, like most other mammals, are commonly affected by various abnormal skin conditions. The causes vary widely and may result from the following: parasitic dermatitis, feed allergies, contact allergies, ringworm, warts, skin tumors, solar dermatitis, prolonged moisture dermatitis, dermatitis from nutritional deficiencies, and unknown causes.

Parasitic Dermatitis

Parasitic dermatitis can be caused by a number of different parasites, but lice and ticks are the most common. Mange mites may also be common in some areas. In my experience, lice and ticks are mainly problems in the winter.

Lice

Signs. Lice suck blood and cause a generalized *intense itching.* Affected horses will rub up against trees, fences, or any convenient object. The mane, tail, and back areas are most affected. Adult lice are large enough to see but because they are small, they frequently are not seen. Small, cream-colored nits or eggs may frequently be found under the hairs of the mane.

Procedure. Bathing with a good insecticide, properly diluted, is the most effective means of treatment. Old sheep dip-like preparations are not very effective and cause skin irritation to the horse. Because lice are always a herd problem, all horses running together should be done the same day. If the weather is too cold for bathing, suitable lice powder preparations should be applied until the weather permits bathing. The bathing should be repeated in 3 weeks in order to kill the new adults that have developed from the nits or eggs which were not killed by the first treatment. A proper insecticide should be recommended by a veterinarian.

Ticks

Signs. Ticks most often will be found in scattered locations on the body. They may occur along the neck and over the back, but they often prefer being inside the thighs of the back legs. The female ticks become larger than the males as they become engorged with blood. Ticks can spread diseases and may occur in such large numbers as to cause acute anemia, which can result in the death of the animal if it is only slightly stressed in its acute anemic condition.

Procedure. Control is difficult, but affected animals can be effectively treated by bathing with a proper insecticide. Individual ticks can be forcibly picked off with very little concern about the tick's head remaining buried in the skin and causing further problems.

Insect Bites

Signs. Occasionally, mosquito bites or bee stings can cause temporary local swellings, but these usually subside after a short period of time (12 to 24 hours).

Procedure. Antihistamines or cortisone drugs are effective. The use of 8 to 10 Dristan or other suitable antihistamine tablets crushed and given in the grain morning and evening for three treatments usually alleviates the problem. Acute allergic reactions should be treated by a veterinarian.

Onchocerciasis

This is a skin condition of horses that is characterized by blotchy loss of hair on the side of the neck (often down to the shoulder), face, and along the ventral abdomen (the midline of the belly wall). Many black horses will take on a "polkadot" appearance. Itching is not a symptom and, if it occurs, is not severe.

Cause. The small hairlike worm called Onchocera cervicalis is the cause and has been shown to be a parasite that affects the majority of horses in many parts of the world. The larvae of this parasite are called microfilariae and they frequently migrate into the eye as well as to the skin. The skin irritation is believed to be a hypersensitivity to the microfilariae that die during their tissue migration or just to their presence.

Symptoms. A blotchy dermatitis that commonly involves the head, neck, and ventral abdomen. Most active cases are observed during the warm months of the year, though some authorities don't consider this a seasonal disease. Some scurfiness in the affected areas is usually observed.

Treatment. There is no known effective way to prevent this parasite from affecting individual horses. This dermatitis is not contagious. The skin is treated with a therapeutic dandruff shampoo. Good results have been achieved by using a drug called diethylcarbamazine to kill the microfilariae, which is given orally for 21 days. The worm medication, Ivermectin, may be effective. The use of corticosteroids with antibiotics might also be indicated if any open lesions are present or if much itching is noted. Periodic retreatment may be necessary.

Ear Plaques

This is a skin condition of the horse that is observed throughout the United States. It is characterized by multiple grayish white circular lesions inside the ears. It occurs in all breeds, although it is almost nonexistent in horses less than 1 year old.

Cause. The exact cause is not known, but it is believed to be a tissue reaction to the biting of the black flies (Similium spp.), which can be found feeding on the inner ears during the summer. Droplets of blood and dried blood are often observed. Attempts to isolate a pathogenic fungus have not been successful.

Symptoms. Inside the ears, there are several grayish white crusty plaques (round slightly raised circles) that often have the appearance of battery corrosion. The crustiness can easily be rubbed off. Underneath may or may not be an irritated raw lesion. Such a lesion is most likely an irritation from the biting rather than from the crusty material. Horses are often irritated by these biting insects, and ear flicking or rubbing is common. Even though these plaques as such are not normally seen in horses under a year, the author has observed blood droplets from the bites of these black flies in the ears of newborn foals less than 24 hours old. It should be noted that similar symptoms can be caused by ear ticks.

Treatment. Cutting the hair out of the ears, as in grooming for a show, can be helpful in reducing the biting of these flies, which normally rest on these hairs between "meals." An antibiotic-cortisone ointment is usually helpful in reducing the local irritation, but once the plaques are present, they most likely will remain. They seem to cause no irritation or problem. The use of a fly repellent gel can be very useful as a preventative measure.

Vetch Hay Allergy

Nutritionally, vetch hay is very good for horses, but many horses will show an allergic response to it (Figs. 109 and 110).

Signs

Geldings that are allergic to vetch hay characteristically develop a *swollen sheath*, which may become very large and appear to interfere with urination (Fig. 111). This is seldom the case; urine is usually still able to escape from the swollen sheath despite the fact that the swelling may interfere with the extension of the penis from the sheath. Mares commonly develop a *swollen udder* and may appear to have milk. Some owners mistakenly think the mare is in foal and are concerned about having her examined for pregnancy. Vetch in any stage of growth can cause this allergic response in the horse. While growing in the pasture, it has a blue to purple bloom. It is often referred to as a "wild pea" as pods develop. Finding the dried blossoms and the pods and the characteristic leaf structure in the hay confirms the diagnosis.

Procedure

Severe cases best respond to injection of cortisone-type drugs, but oral antihistamines are often effective. The source of the vetch must be removed. Ten 5-grain aspirins in the grain are also helpful.

Feed Bumps

These are multiple small skin swellings that are caused by various plants. Most often it represents an allergic response of individual horses to certain plants. This occasionally occurs from the feeding of certain prepared feeds. Grain mixtures high in linseed meal are common offenders. When they occur on horses in pasture, they are referred to simply as "pasture bumps."

Signs

Multiple small skin eruptions will be observed over the horse's body, mostly over the neck, back, and croup. A small amount of serum will have leaked out of the skin causing the bumps to have a small scab or to be crusty.

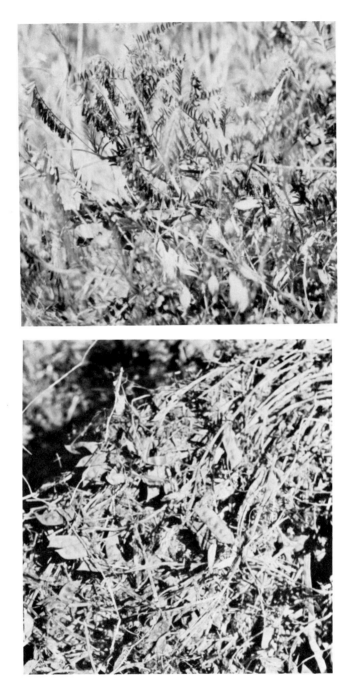

FIGS. 109 and 110.   Vetch is good nutritionally, but horses commonly develop allergies to it.

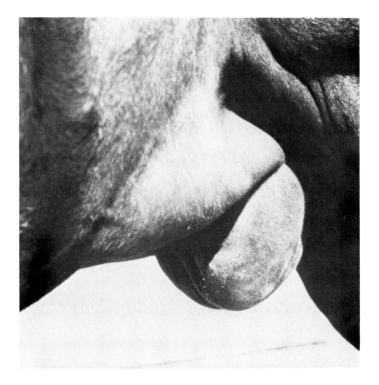

FIG. 111.   Swollen sheaths or udders are symptoms of vetch allergies.

Procedure

Of primary concern is elimination of the cause. Many times these symptoms are brought on only by certain growth stages of plants and horses may continue to be in a pasture and have the lesions disappear and not recur. During the active stages, bathing with tincture of green soap and the giving of antihistamines or aspirin in the grain can be effective.

Allergic Dermatitis

This is an annually recurring seasonal disease that is characterized by acute itching along the mane and tail of horses during the warmer summer months. Occasionally most of the body may be affected. This condition occurs widely throughout the world and is known by such names as "Queensland itch," "sweet itch," and "allergic urticaria" (Fig. 111A).

Cause

It is believed to be the result of individual horses being hypersensitive to the saliva of certain biting insects. The mosquito,

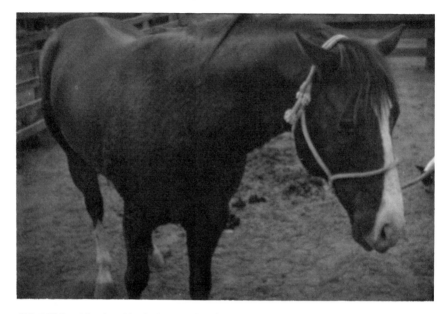

FIG. 111A.   Allergic urticaria from a plant in some new hay.

Aedes triseriatus, and the small gnat-like insect (midge) night feeder, Culicoides variiepennis, have been incriminated, but other species might also be involved. It has been thought that the microfilariae of Onchocera cervicalis might also be a causative factor, but it now appears that the condition is the result of sensitivity to the bites of various insects. A similar disease occurs in dogs that are allergic to fleas.

Incidence

This allergic dermatitis is first noticed in the late spring or early summer and often continues to be a problem until the cold weather comes. This period corresponds to the peak of the insect season.

Symptoms

The primary symptom is an intense itching. Lice need to be eliminated as the possible cause. An affected animal often rubs its mane and neck under a branch or board of a fence or its hind quarters and tail against a post, fence, or tree. Open lesions often develop from its rubbing against these objects. A blotchy loss of hair is frequently noticed around the face. Though the condition is an allergic reaction, the skin usually develops an itching reaction with or without scurf. The marked leaking out of serum and crusty lesions as seen from tick bites and solar dermatitis is not common, though it does occasionally occur.

It should be noted that there is evidence that there may be a potential inherited susceptibility to this condition, which is not uncommon with many allergies observed among lower animals and man.

Treatment

Treatment is aimed at reducing the irritation from both an external and internal approach. Bathing with tincture of green soap or any mild soap followed by a therapeutic shampoo prescribed by a veterinarian. This is lathered up and left on for 10 to 15 minutes and then rinsed well. This is usually repeated in 4 or 5 days. Injections of corticosteroids with antibiotics are usually given to initially control the itching and to treat open infections of local lesions. Oral corticosteroids or aspirin can be temporarily effective. The use of insecticide sprays may also be useful. Since the midge rarely begins feeding before 4:30 PM and rarely enters buildings, the stabling of affected animals in a shelter during the late day and night, when biting insects are the most active, has proven quite helpful and often curative. The condition commonly disappears as early as 3 to 4 weeks after affected horses are sheltered this way. During the winter months, the skin of affected animals usually returns to normal.

Contact Allergies

Most such allergies are the result of contact with insecticides or fly repellents not properly diluted. Oil-base products are the most common offenders.

Signs

The area where the insecticide was applied will appear slightly elevated or swollen and sensitive. It may or may not develop a crusty appearance, depending on the severity of the irritation and whether it caused serum to escape from the affected skin.

Procedure

Clean area thoroughly with soap (tincture of green soap works well) and water to remove any insecticide residue. Oral antihistamines and cortisone-like drugs are indicated and helpful.

Prolonged Moisture Dermatitis

Signs

Excess moisture on the skin can cause problems. When the *feet* are in mud or other wet conditions for a long time, they develop an equivalent condition to "dish pan hands." The outer wall of the hooves becomes soft and the area directly below the coronary band of the hooves sheds a thin whitish outer layer of the wall. The heels become very soft and may develop a tenderness. The skin of the pastern may become actively inflamed. If the *skin* goes for a long period (2 weeks or more) without getting a chance to dry out, it may develop a scurfiness under the hair which in turn falls out (Fig. 112). This is equivalent to "wool rot" in sheep. The croup area is the most affected, but sometimes the mane will also be affected.

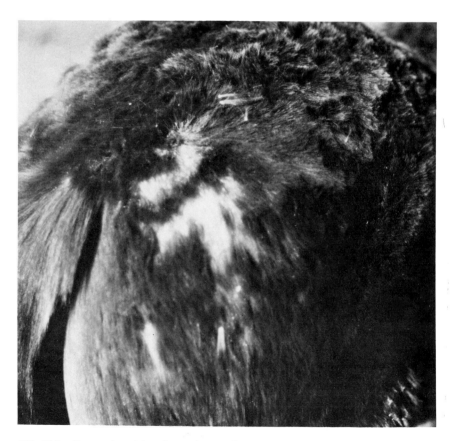

FIG. 112.   Too much moisture from rainy weather can cause hair loss.

Procedure

Bathe with tincture of green soap or other therapeutic shampoo, groom well, and allow the animal to dry out. Try to get the animal out of the mud. Building a large (30 × 30 feet) feeding area such as a slightly elevated platform is recommended for horses in pastures during the winter. An inexpensive platform can be made by laying down old railroad ties very close together over the area desired. Sand is then poured over the ties. The sand fills into the cracks between the ties, thus making an elevated area with good drainage on which to feed. This gives the animals a place out of the mud during the winter.

In cases of acute "mud fever," where there are swollen legs, actively inflamed skin in the pastern areas, and marked tenderness (Figs. 113 and 114), one should remove the animal from mud to a stall or well-drained area; thoroughly clean the affected legs with soap and warm water; bandage the legs using nitrofurazone or antibiotic dressing, changing bandages daily until the condition is under control; and use aspirin to reduce swelling and inflammation (10 aspirin twice daily in grain).

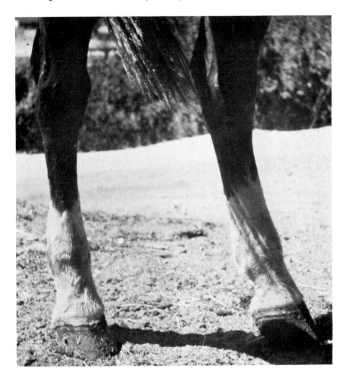

FIG. 113.   If mud is allowed to remain on the skin of the legs for a long period "mud fever" can occur.

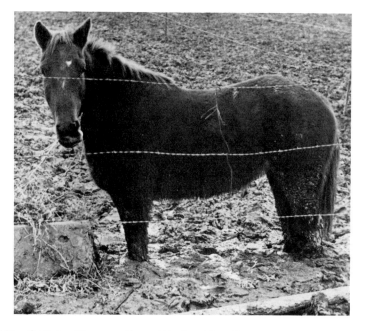

FIG. 114.   Such conditions usually result in "mud fever."

Solar Dermatitis (Sun Burn)

Signs

This particular skin condition is the result of an animal developing photosensitization. Certain plants may contain a photodynamic agent which can cause a problem in some sensitive individual horses. When this agent—which is ingested and gets into the blood stream—is circulating close to the skin surface in white, unpigmented areas, it absorbs sun rays. These rays then cause a typical sun-burning effect to the skin, from mild scruffing to large areas of dead skin peeling away. A seriously affected animal, such as a pinto, may have very large white areas on the body dry up, become hard, and peel. The lesions are characteristically restricted to the white areas, being very common on the muzzles of blaze-faced horses.

Procedure

Such horses are best removed from the offending pasture and kept in the dark until the agent is metabolized out of the body— which may be up to 5 to 7 days. Minor skin irritations can be effectively treated with common suntan lotions. Severe cases should be under the care of a veterinarian and may require the administration of anti-inflammatory drugs and antibiotics.

Nonspecific Dermatitis

Signs

There are, as has been discussed, many different causes of skin conditions in the horse. Besides the specific causes already mentioned, nutritional deficiencies, especially vitamin A, and heavy internal parasitism can be important underlying causes. Many cases go undiagnosed. A common nonspecific sign may be blotchy loss of hair around the face or other areas on the body, which is not accompanied by itching (Fig. 115).

Procedure

An effective general treatment for many skin conditions is the bathing of the horse with tincture of green soap, followed by a

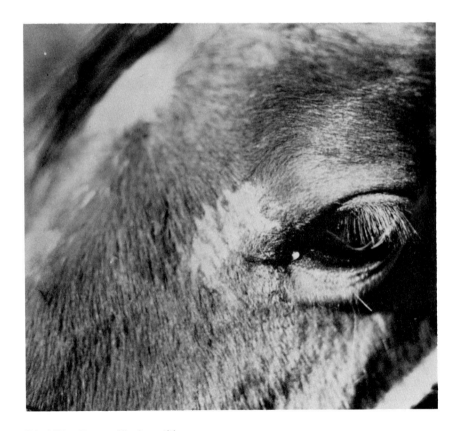

FIG. 115. Nonspecific dermatitis.

rinse in a safe, prescribed insecticide, such as might be used for lice.[13] Contact your veterinarian for specific recommendations.

Ringworm

This condition is caused by a fungus and usually affects young, debilitated animals, but may affect any horse. The condition is potentially highly contagious to other horses but only very mildly contagious to man.

Signs

Dry, scaly, encrusted round lesions with loss of hair will appear most commonly on the skin around the eyes, muzzle, saddle girth area, and various other parts of the body (Fig. 116).

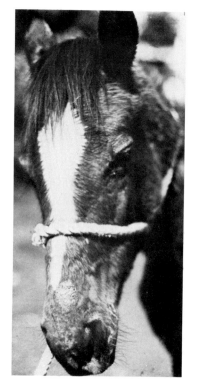

FIG. 116.   Ringworm is a fungus that usually occurs around the face but may occur elsewhere on the body.

---

[13]Always follow dilution instructions carefully when using an insecticide. It is best to avoid oil-based products for use on the horse. Many therapeutic skin shampoos are also available (e.g., Selsun Blue).

Procedure

Modern fungicide creams and shampoos are very effective such as Tinactin cream and Selsun Blue shampoo. Consistent treatment for 4 to 7 days followed by a similar treatment period a week later is often necessary to effectively treat this type of fungus condition.

Warts

Warts are small skin tumors that are caused by a virus. They occur on most mammals throughout the world (Fig. 117). Warts from one species do not appear to spread to other animals. Biting insects may play a part in spreading the virus, as can direct contact.

Signs

The small growths mostly affect young horses and occur around the muzzle area. They may be few in number or numerous. The warts are unsightly, but seldom cause any problem.

Procedure

Warts usually disappear without any treatment in 2 to 6 months. They always go away. Occasionally, the application of the twitch will cause some warts to be knocked off. In the process, some of the virus can be taken into the blood stream of the animal. This frequently stimulates an immune response which can shorten the duration of the disease. The daily application of castor oil to the warts may be helpful. "Tincture of time" is a guaranteed cure.

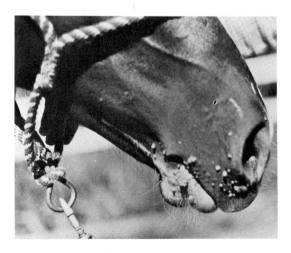

FIG. 117. Warts are caused by a virus. They always go away in time.

Neoplasms

Tumors, which are abnormal tissue growths, are not uncommon on the horse. The noncancerous (benign) tumors rarely cause a problem but are usually removed for aesthetic reasons. The two most common cancerous (malignant) tumors of horses are squamous cell carcinomas and malignant melanomas.

Signs

Squamous cell carcinomas most commonly occur on the penis or around or on the eyes of horses that have little or no pigmentation around their eyes, such as albinos and Appaloosas (Fig. 118). They appear as raw, red granulation tissue. Malignant melanomas are mostly found on gray horses. These are abnormal black tissue growths. They usually occur around the anus or vulva, under the tail, and in the mouth region (Fig. 119).

Procedure

Early cases of carcinomas can be effectively treated with strontium-90 probes or small stylets of strontium-90 injected into the cancer. Most recently available is a drug called Ribigen, which is

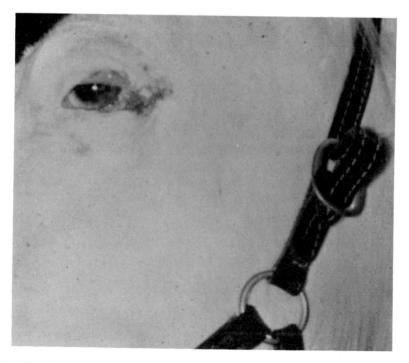

FIG. 118.   Squamous cell carcinomas most often affect the eye area of white horses.

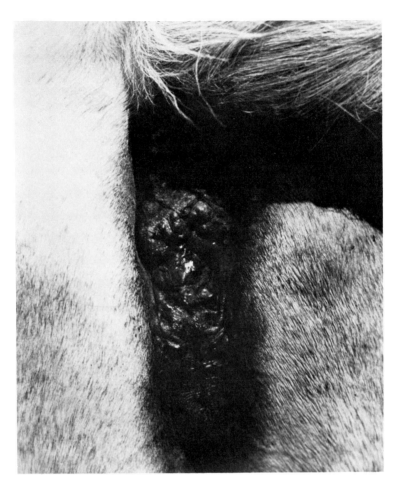

FIG. 119. Malignant melanomas usually occur around the vulva of gray mares.

injected directly into the cancer and is very effective. It is a break-
through in cancer treatment. Surgery is necessary for more advanced cases. Surgery is only of value for early cases of malignant
melanomas; the tumor has a tendency to spread rapidly in a given
area and the condition soon becomes inoperable. Where carcinomas on the penis may spread relatively rapidly (2 to 6 months)
into the body, the other forms may take years to cause problems
from invasion of internal tissues. Horses almost always live a full
life even with melanomas.

Equine Sarcoids

Sarcoids are fairly common skin tumors of the horse. They usually appear on the side of the neck, on the head or ears, and occasionally on the legs. They are thought to be caused by a virus but they do not regress spontaneously. When surgically removed they frequently recur. Cryosurgery (freezing) has been effective but now Ribigen, as for squamous cell carcinomas, is proving very effective, injected directly into the tumor itself. When left untreated they commonly become raw and are unsightly.

INTERNAL DISORDERS

Excess Salivation

The most common causes of excess salivation in the horse are irritation from foxtails, other weeds, or bearded barley; a stick caught and jammed across the palate between the upper chewing teeth; chemical burns, such as from nosing into the lime used to dry and disinfect stall floors; and bad teeth or a severe bit irritation or damage to the tissues of the mouth. Once the cause has been determined and corrected, the condition clears up. To examine the back area of the mouth for the possible presence of a jammed stick, it is best to hold the mouth open with a dental wedge. A dental wedge can be constructed from a 5 or 6 inch wooden block of a 2 × 4 inch board cut into a wedge shape, and cut in half lengthwise. This should be well sanded to prevent splinters. It is also good to tie a small diameter rope to it for easier removal. This is jammed back on one side of the mouth while the palate area is examined. Extra vitamin A and B supplements help mouth-wound healing. It is good to remove foxtails mechanically from mouth wounds.

Diarrhea in the Horse

Diarrhea in the adult horse is usually the result of inflammation in the intestinal tract (enteritis). Internal parasites (worms), moldy hay, allergic response to a feed (walnut leaves are a common cause), occasionally a protozoan (micro-organism) infection, and even a heavy infestation of lice can cause diarrhea in the horse. If severe diarrhea occurs, causing very watery manure, signs of spasmodic colic often occur. The horse may become very colicky with many signs of distress—sweating, kicking at its abdomen, and rolling—with the intermittent passage of very loose manure. Such animals should receive veterinary care.

Treatment

Remove and eliminate the cause if it can be determined. The use of a broad-spectrum antibiotic intravenously is usually very helpful; there is almost always some degree of an intestinal infection. Specific problems need specific treatment and severe or prolonged cases should receive veterinary attention. The use of aspirin (ten 5-grain tablets), with or without a bran mash, is helpful. A bran mash with the aspirin and 2 tablespoons of baking soda is soothing to the inflamed tissues.[14] In general, it is good for the animal to be placed on a good, clean oat or timothy hay diet for a few days.

Constipation

Constipation in the adult horse is more common in the aged animal, though it may occur at any age. Such horses may pass only small amounts of firm, possibly mucous-covered, manure. More advanced cases can develop into complete blockage and show typical signs of colic. Sudden changes in feed, gorging of grain, intestinal tract damage from worms, graining an overheated animal, feeding too much of finely ground grain or mixture, eating off a sandy ground, an aged and less active digestive tract, and poor teeth can all be potential causes.

Treatment

If complete blockage seems evident, a veterinarian should be called as soon as possible. A bran mash may be helpful in early, mild cases. It is always potentially dangerous to drench a horse with any large quantity of fluid, especially with mineral oil, which can easily get into the lungs. Milk of magnesia (16 ounces) is less dangerous and is effective. The routine giving of a bran mash twice weekly to older horses is often good preventive medicine.

Shivering

Shivering is nature's way to physiologically stimulate circulation to help increase body temperature. The most common cause is chilling that has resulted from exposure in cold rains and cold weather. Shivering also can result as a secondary symptom of shock or pain.

If cold weather is the cause, it is desirable to bring the animal into a barn or shelter, rub it dry, blanket it, and fix it a hot bran

---

[14]If the horse is too uncomfortable to take the aspirin in a bran mash, it is possible to give it by crushing it up and mixing it with honey and then gobbing this into the corner of the horse's mouth.

mash. If the animal is in good health and no shelter is available, a hot bran mash alone helps to warm it up. A grain ration of one-quarter cracked corn is also helpful to the horse in cold weather.

If shivering is secondary to shock or pain, the medical cause should be treated by a veterinarian, but blanketing and the offering of a hot bran mash are safe procedures. The bran mash should never be force fed.

13

Injuries and Treatments

Horses, in general, are accident-prone and are frequently injured. This can be attributed to two basic causes: (1) horses by nature run when frightened, and (2) man frequently provides an unsafe environment for the horse (e.g., protruding nails and bolts, barbed-wire fences, junk-cluttered areas). Man subjects these animals to undue stress, (e.g., 2-year-old racing, unreasonable endurance tests and riding courses, very high jumping, and rodeo activities). In basic good horsemanship, one should be able to recognize situations that are most likely to cause injuries and take steps to avoid and prevent those situations from occurring.

Common Situations that Result in Injuries

Poor stabling conditions include:
1. Protruding nails and bolts
2. Barbed-wire fences and fences in bad repair
3. Uncapped steel fence posts
4. Old farm equipment, abandoned cars, and miscellaneous junk in area
5. Jagged points on feed and water containers
6. Too-small stable area allowing a horse to be cast in stall or barn
7. Inadequate bedding on floor of stall
8. Poorly secured locks on gates or grain room

Poor husbandry procedures include:
1. Overcrowding and not allowing new horses an acquaintance period while being separated by a fence

2. Not separating very aggressive horses that are likely to injure others
3. Not allowing ample area between horses when feeding
4. Hanging feed or water containers from fences or walls with wire and leaving ends of wire exposed
5. Turning horses out into new surroundings at night, especially with strange horses
6. Working with animals under low overhangs
7. Improper methods of tying horses
8. Allowing mares to foal with other horses
9. Not providing safe area for foaling
10. Overworking and exposure to undue stress

INFLAMMATION

All injuries cause inflammation. Nature has provided all animals with a mechanism to respond to an injury so that healing can occur. It is imperative that one treating such conditions have a basic understanding of the process of inflammation, what it is, its causes and results.

Classically, there are four signs of inflammation: *swelling, heat, pain,* and *redness.* Due to the pigmentation of animals' skin, redness is not normally observed. When an injury occurs, some local cells are damaged and these damaged cells release chemicals that stimulate the inflammatory process. This results in an increased blood circulation in the area, an increased dilation and permeability of the blood vessels to allow serum and defense-type blood cells to dilute the irritant, localize its effect, and destroy it. In the process, swelling occurs from the increased fluid in the area of injured tissues and this presses on local nerve endings resulting in pain. The object of the pain is to cause the animal to be aware of the injury so the area will be moved as little as possible in order for healing to occur. The increased circulation to the area brings more blood to the surface and accounts for the heat. It should be noted that most often only very acute inflammation results in a detectable increase in local heat over an injured area. It is often very difficult to distinguish increased local heat from that which is normal. An increased, strong pounding pulse (digital pulse) in the feet is very helpful in clinically detecting inflammation in the hooves.

Treatment of Inflammation

Although nature's way is often very effective, the inflammatory process frequently results in a prolonged healing period. Excessive swelling can actually cause additional damage to the area.

It is now known that a shorter healing period can be accomplished if attempts are made to minimize the initial inflammation resulting from an injury. If this is done, we must accompany the treatment with *forced rest* and protection against infection by the *use of antibiotics* if a wound has occurred. To markedly reduce inflammation is to not allow the body to muster its forces against infection and irritants.

There are basically two types of inflammation—"acute" and "chronic." Most relatively nonsevere injuries will go through an immediate period of acute inflammation followed by rapid healing, if there are no complications. The recovery period is relatively short—1 to 4 weeks. After this period, the animal can be returned to normal activity. More severe injuries also go through an initial period of acute inflammation, but as this period subsides, often there occurs a slower, prolonged chronic inflammation period. This period may extend over several months before the horse is fully recovered.

Treatment of Acute Inflammation

Cold is always applied to an initial injury to constrict local blood vessels and minimize swelling. Early application of heat can cause a "blow up" reaction causing more swelling by relaxing local vessels and thus worsening the condition. The only use of heat in early treatments is in the attempt to establish drainage in a foot puncture wound, to bring an abscess to a head, or in cases of minor muscle strain. Always remember the rule that for *early treatment* of an injury, "cold is safe, hot is not." It should be noted, also, that the early application of heat to a foot that has been injured from kicking out and hitting a stall wall or other solid object can contribute to the quick building up of calcium deposit in the pastern area, which forms a ringbone condition.

Cold Application. Cold application methods include: (1) holding or securing under a bandage a plastic bag of crushed ice; (2) use of an ice boot, pant leg, or inner tube with ice; (3) cold stream of water from a hose (duration of treatments is 10 to 20 minutes once or twice daily); and (4) standing horse in mud up over the coronary bands (hairline) for 2 hours daily.

Heat Applications. To help establish drainage in hoof puncture wounds, soak foot in plastic bucket of water (not too hot for the hand) into which is dissolved 2 cups of epsom salts. Soak the foot 15 to 20 minutes once or twice daily for 4 days. It should be noted that surgical drainage may be necessary.

Hot compresses applied to an abscess help it come to a head for lancing. Soak a face towel in hot epsom salts water (2 cups in 1 gallon of water). Epsom salts creates some drawing action but mostly helps keep the water warm longer. Ring towel out and hold it on the area until towel cools. Then rewet the towel and reapply it to the area. Continue this process for 15 to 20 minutes, once or twice daily. Wrapping the hot towel in aluminum foil keeps it warm longer. Running hot water on to the area is effective, as is the use of whirlpools. Ichthammol ointment or other poultices such as hot medicated poultice, epsom salts paste, or bran applied daily also have a drawing effect. They work by providing continuous heat.

Treatment with Drugs. Chemical treatments for inflammation are very effective and can greatly help reduce acute inflammation. In centuries past, horses were bled to reduce blood pressure in the hooves in cases of laminitis. Today, we have a greater understanding of the physiology involved and such radical procedures are neither necessary nor indicated.

Aspirin is not widely known to have an effective anti-inflammatory action. Its use is indicated for the treatment of any inflammation in the horse where tissue swelling or pain is present. Harmful effects have not been noted. The usual dose is 10 (5 grains) tablets, dissolved in a little water mixed in the grain twice daily—that is 20 tablets a day for a 1000-pound animal. Give smaller dosage to smaller horses (e.g., 5 tablets for 500-pound animal). The inexpensive aspirin works just as well as the more expensive brands.

Cortisone-related drugs have marked anti-inflammatory actions but should only be used by a veterinarian. These drugs can work miracles in the early treatment of joint, muscle, and tendon injuries. Since they can lower the body's defense mechanisms against infections, their use in the face of a wound or infection should always be accompanied with the use of broad-spectrum antibiotics.

Phenylbutazone is an effective analgesic (pain reducer) as well as an anti-inflammatory agent. The use of any pain killer can mask the seriousness of an injury. Sufficient time and rest are always needed for an injury to heal. Working animals too soon after an injury, especially with the use of an analgesic, can predispose the animal to further tissue damage and perhaps more serious injury. This drug should only be used under the prescription of a veterinarian.

Dimethyl sulfoxide (DMSO) is a chemical solution that is a by-product of the paper mill industry and has been found to have an anti-inflammatory effect when applied locally to an acute swelling resulting from an injury. It has also sometimes been found effective when applied to more chronic conditions such as splints, ringbone, or other bony enlargements, but no one treatment has yet offered consistent favorable results for these conditions. This product should only be used under the close guidance of a veterinarian.

Orgotein is a chemical obtained from the liver of cattle. It has a broad-based anti-inflammatory effect when given as an injection to horses and other animals. It is reported to have had a high degree of success in the treatment of such chronic equine disorders as osselets, joint inflammations, ringbone, sidebone, laminitis, bursitis, and ligament problems. It is available for commercial use but is expensive. Its long-term effects have yet to be evaluated.

Treatment of Chronic Inflammation

Many cases of chronic inflammation can be effectively treated with cortisone-related drugs injected directly into the affected area, along with time and good nursing. Years ago, it was found that many cases could be treated by purposely causing acute inflammation to the affected area, which would result in a faster recovery period—the idea being that the renewed increased circulation to the injured area would bring about a faster repair of the damaged tissue. This is the theory behind counter irritation.

Counter Irritation

Counter irritation can be achieved by a complete range of medicinal and physical procedures. The progression of severity is as follows: liniments, sweats, leg paints, blisters, and firing.

Firing is the strongest form of counter-irritant treatment. This is the application of a hot welding-like iron with a fine point to an anesthetized leg or area in the pattern of a series of puncture dots. The overall effectiveness of this procedure is questioned by many veterinarians and horsemen. Many equine veterinarians feel that better results can be achieved by the early use of anti-inflammatory drugs, proper immobilization or supportive bandages, flexocasts or plaster casts, and sufficient time for rest. It has often been said that the best place to fire a horse is where the saddle sits—thus giving the horse a forced rest period. It should be clearly understood that the counter-irritant treatment is not constructive in any sense of the word. In fact, it is destructive in nature. It does not strengthen—it weakens. Anti-inflammatory drugs, good nursing, and *time* are felt by many to be the method of choice even in the treatment of chronic inflammation. The effects of the severe forms of counter irritation such as blistering and firing can be rightfully challenged on the basis of being inhumane.

WOUND TREATMENT CHART

WOUNDS & INJURIES	MEDICATION & TREATMENT RECOMMENDED	MEDICATION NOT TO USE
MINOR SCRAPE or ABRASIONS	Nitrofurazone (yellow) spray	Salves
MINOR SKIN SCRATCHES	Same as above	Salves
ROPE BURN—Superficial	Same as above	Salves
*ROPE BURN—Deep	Nitrofurazone salve under bandage	Astringents or Caustics
SMALL SKIN WOUND—left open	Nitrofurazone spray or powder	Astringents or Caustics
*LARGE SKIN WOUND—to be sutured	Nitrofurazone salve under bandage	Astringents or Caustics
*LARGE SKIN WOUND—left open	Nitrofurazone spray	Astringents or Caustics
*JAGGED SKIN WOUND—to be sutured	Nitrofurazone salve under bandage; Nitrofurazone powder if not able to bandage	Astringents or Caustics
*JAGGED DEEP MUSCLE WOUND—to be sutured	Same as above	Astringents or Caustics
*DEEP OPEN WOUND—over 48 hrs. old	Nitrofurazone spray or powder	Astringents or Caustics
OPEN WOUND—healed to skin level	Same as above	Astringents or Caustics
*OPEN WOUND—with "proud flesh"	Neo-predef powder; trim flat, if necessary	Tissue, stimulants
*PUNCTURE WOUND—in soft tissue	Nitrofurazone spray or powder	Astringents or Caustics
*PUNCTURE WOUND—in hoof	Tincture of iodine, Betadine, or Kopertox; plug with cotton	Caustics
MINOR WOUND To HOOF CORONARY BAND	Kopertox or Nitrofurazone spray	Caustics
MINOR SPRAIN or SWOLLEN LEG	Same as above	Heat Applications, e.g. Liniments, Sweats, Leg Paints or Blisters

*Such wounds should be under the care of a veterinarian.

GENERAL INITIAL TREATMENT INDICATED FOR ALL WOUNDS:

1. Control bleeding by direct pressure as needed.
2. Trim hair from wound margins.
3. Clean with only mild soap and water; rinse well
4. Dead tissue should be removed as necessary
5. Suture if possible
6. Proper wound dressing application

7. Tetanus Protection
8. Administration of Antibiotics as needed
9. Bandage if possible
10. Aspirin in grain twice daily to minimize tissue swelling
11. Fly repellant around wound as needed
12. Restricted movement in a clean stall or small paddock as needed

NOTES: 1. After initial treatment, try to keep wounds as clean and dry as possible, avoid frequent washings.
2. Salves should not be applied to open wounds as they collect dirt and debris.
3. Wounds should be sutured within first 12 hours, but often are still suturable from 24 to 36 hours depending upon tissue swelling and blood supply to injured skin.
4. Neo-predef powder is a neomycin-cortisone product by Upjohn.
5. Amway's L.O.C. is a mild soap and very good for cleaning wounds; it is not irritating to the tissues.

WOUNDS

The seriousness of a wound varies greatly and depends on the following factors: the depth of the injury, the amount of tissue damaged, its location, and the nature of the tissue affected. Obviously, deep jagged wounds into important structures such as joints, tendons, and eyes are more serious than superficial wounds or those into muscle areas. Because serious wounds can result in permanent disability, unsoundness, or death, all such wounds should receive prompt veterinary care for proper treatment. Many less severe wounds can be treated by the owner if the owner understands the basic principles of wound treatments. He must also realize that each type of wound—and wounds at different stages of healing—require different treatment procedures and medications. The following guidelines are helpful in providing for proper wound treatment.

Wound Care

The Don'ts of Wound Treatment

1. Don't apply any astringent or caustic, such as gentian violet, tincture of iodine, copper sulfate, or alum to any fresh wound more severe than a superficial scrape, abrasion, or scratch.
2. Don't apply *any* medicine to a wound that will need to be sutured unless it is recommended by a veterinarian to be used as a first-aid until he arrives. Washing it with a mild soap and water is safe. The use of peroxide can be irritating to the tissues and it should not be used in a wound to be sutured.
3. Don't apply a salve, such as petroleum jelly, corona, or nitrofurazone, to any *open* wound; this accumulates dirt and debris.
4. Don't wash a wound frequently with water, peroxide, or *any* liquid; this slows healing and stimulates the growth of proud flesh. Horse's tissues "waterlog" very easily.
5. Don't wrap a leg without good padding under the bandage; this can cut into the leg or restrict blood circulation. This is especially true in young foals.
6. Don't leave a stretch bandage on more than 24 hours. Daily removal is necessary to ensure proper circulation. Vetraps, though, are safe over a prolonged period of time, such as 5 to 7 days, as necessary.
7. Don't use sugar or salt water in the eyes. Fresh water or boric acid rinses are safe.

General Treatment Procedures for New Wounds

1. *Clean wounds* thoroughly with mild soap and water, removing all dirt and foreign matter. Do not use peroxide or irritating disinfectant or cleaning agent. These cause further tissue damage and will slow healing. Shave surrounding hair. Avoid frequent use of water in future care, horse's tissues seem to "waterlog" very easily; this also will tend to slow healing and stimulate excess granulation tissue. Use clean gauze pads or cloth to remove debris after initial cleaning.
2. *Control bleeding* by direct pressure with a pad of cloth (e.g., 4-inch-square face cloth) over the wound, either held in place with a tight bandage well padded or by holding in place firmly until the veterinarian arrives if the wound is in an area that cannot be bandaged. Use of tourniquets is never needed; even the most severe bleeding can be controlled by direct pressure. If excess bleeding is coming from large puncture area, pack an unrolled clean gauze or cloth deep into the wound. If nitrofurazone salve or liquid is available, place some of this on the packing. If not, do not use any medicine that is likely to cause further tissue damage.
3. *Immobilize the wound* if possible. Suturing helps speed healing and minimizes scar formation. Injuries to eyelids should always be sutured if possible to avoid future drying of the eye. Wounds are best sutured within 12 to 24 hours. If the wound is over a joint or in an area where extensive movement occurs, the horse should be stalled and only allowed controlled exercise. The use of a flexible cast or plaster cast may be indicated. The use of a cradle (a necklace device that prevents the horse's head from contacting its chest or front legs) may be necessary to prevent an animal from removing front-leg bandages or chewing at wounds on the legs or chest. Routine use of aspirin following injuries minimizes wound itching and keeps down tissue swelling; sutures are commonly left in for approximately 3 weeks to prevent accidental reopening of the wound (Fig. 120).
4. *Prevent infection* by local application of an antibacterial dressing and by administering systemic antibiotics. Always use non-irritating wound dressings in deep wounds, bandaging when possible. The initial use of astringents or caustics kills the top layer of cells, which then must slough out during the healing process. They not only slow early healing but also make it almost impossible to refreshen and suture a wound that has been so treated (Fig. 121).
5. *Tetanus protection* should be considered for *all* wounds be-

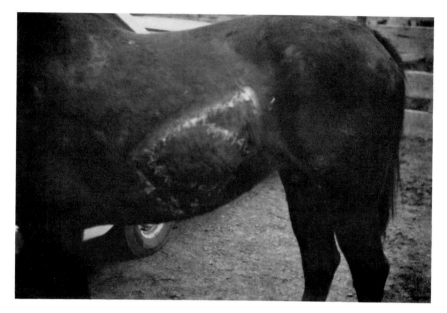

FIG. 120.   Sutured wound.

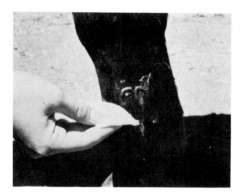

FIG. 121.   Applying nitrofurazone to a wound to be bandaged.

cause the horse is very susceptible to this disease. Tetanus
antitoxin is given to horses not previously vaccinated against
tetanus, whereas other horses that have been through the
series of two tetanus toxoid vaccinations (2 to 8 weeks apart)
are given a tetanus toxoid booster if they have not had a
booster in the last 8 to 12 months.[15]

6. *Bandaging* is helpful to protect wounds from dirt or other

---

[15]Though deep puncture wounds are most often the source for tetanus, occasionally the
disease results from relatively superficial cuts.

irritation and may serve to restrict local tissue movement. Normally, the bandage is changed the second day after the initial treatment and then only every other day. Wounds with excessive drainage should be changed at least daily. Once a good base to the wound has developed, it can be left open (if the wound is not excessively large and flies are not a major problem). Never bandage around a leg without good padding, such as sheet cotton, clean dish towel, or disposable diapers (Fig. 122). Never wrap rubber elastic bandages (ace-type) tightly, as they very easily might cause too much pressure resulting in noticeable discomfort and possible restriction of blood circulation. It is best not to use rubber elastic bandages of any type, because it is so easy to put them on too tightly. Young horses are made susceptible to skin sloughs by allowing bandages to restrict blood circulation. This is not a problem with Vetraps, which are safe and useful for bandaging wounds.

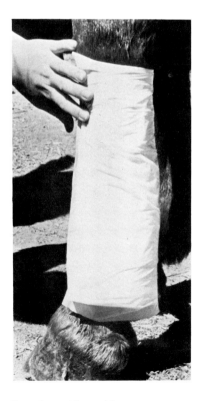

FIG. 122.   A disposable diaper is used for padding.

Restraint Techniques While Treating Wounds

In general, it is best to use as little restraint as possible when working with horses. By working quietly and with no sudden movements, one can often get much accomplished. Treatment of wounds is often a painful experience, so active restraint procedures are indicated and are frequently necessary to make proper treatment possible.

Chemical restraint is very effective. The veterinarian uses injections of tranquilizers, sedatives, or general anesthetics when necessary to treat extensive wounds.

The *twitch* is an extremely helpful tool in the restraint of most horses. It is usually made of a wooden handle, 12 to 24 inches long to which a 12- to 14-inch rope or chain is made into a loop and attached at one end. This loop is placed over the upper lip, not including the nasal cartilage, and is twisted tight, pinching the lip. This pressure causes temporary pain to the nose, which then consumes most of the horse's attention so that other procedures can be carried out. Though this may seem inhumane or cruel, it does most often cause the horse to stand perfectly still and allow the animal to receive proper wound treatment that would otherwise be nearly impossible. Even extensive pressure will not cause any permanent damage to the horse. The use of the twitch on the ear is never recommended because it is possible to cause permanent damage to the cartilage, which will result in constant drooping of the affected ear. (It is important to remember that one must never stand in front of a horse being twitched! Always stay in close to the shoulder or out of striking distance.)

Tying up a front leg with a rope or strap is not recommended; it is easy for the animal to rear up and fall over backward, resulting in serious injury or even death.

Off-balance methods are useful many times when wrapping or applying medicine to a wound. If a front leg is being treated, the other front leg is lifted to force weight on the other legs. If a back leg is being medicated, it is often best to lift the front leg on the same side. This is not necessary, but by having the people handling the horse working on the same side, this can prevent either of them from getting hurt if the animal happens to make any sudden movements of resistance.

Earing a horse just by grabbing it (not biting or twisting it) and using it to physically restrain the horse is often effective and helpful for short temporary restraint. The technique may be very useful when attempting to put a twitch on a resistant patient. Most horses accept the procedure well and do not become persistently ear shy because of its use. Horses with basically resistant temperaments will usually object to any head restraint and will often be leery about being eared.

When restraining a horse, it is best not to have the animal tied and to have plenty of room to move about. Some very wild horses have to be snubbed (tied very close) to a heavy secure post before any restraining techniques can be used. Backing a horse into a corner often makes it easier to work on.

Common Equine Wound Medications[16]

1. Protective salves: vaseline, corona, Bag Balm, lanolin, skin lotions
2. Antiseptics, non-irritating: nitrofurazone solution, salve, powder, and spray, antibiotic ointments, nolvasan salve, povidone-iodine
3. Astringents, irritating and drying to tissues: gentian violet, alum, tincture of iodine
4. Stimulants to tissue growth: scarlet oil, sulfa urea powder, enzyme spray
5. Caustics, treatment for proud flesh: copper sulfate, silver nitrate[17]

Excessive Granulation Tissue (Proud Flesh)[18]

It is normal for wounds to heal by granulating in to fill the space of the damaged tissue. Horses are very prone to produce excessive granulation tissue, which then rises or bulges above the skin surface (Fig. 123). This is especially true in wounds below the knees and the hocks. When this occurs, the edges of the wound are not able to cover this elevated tissue so healing can be completed. This tissue usually becomes larger, protruding high above the level of the skin and bleeds easily when it is bumped. This tissue is raw and red in appearance, has a good blood supply but a very poor nerve supply. When it is much over ¼ inch above the skin level, it is best for it to be surgically removed. Since it has little feeling, this excessive granulation tissue can simply be cut with a scalpel or very sharp knife, causing very little discomfort to the animal. The wound will then bleed fairly freely from the cut small

---

[16]See Chart III for notations on when and when not to use these wound medications. Nitrofurazone solution and powder are safe in any type wound.

[17]More severe caustics should not be used as they cause excessive tissue damage and are usually painful and inhumane.

[18]Excess granulation tissue is stimulated by washing the wound with water too frequently, the daily application of peroxide, use of tissue-stimulating drugs (sulfa urea, scarlet oil, enzyme sprays) after the healing granulation tissue has reached the skin level, and by wood shavings and dirt. It is always best to bed horses with wounds in *straw* rather than shavings and to keep the horse's environment as clean as possible.

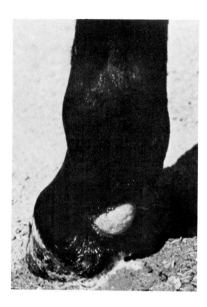

FIG. 123. "Proud flesh" has to be removed before healing can occur.

vessels, but this can easily be controlled with pressure bandaging. The wound is kept bandaged for 2 to 4 days, then left open and treated with neomycin-cortisone powder or caustic powder until it is healed. The use of severe caustics should be avoided for the treatment of this problem.

Eye Injuries

Eye injuries or inflammation should be treated conscientiously to avoid permanent damage. Flush eye well with clean water and examine carefully the degree and nature of the problem. Never use sugar water or salt water to flush out the eyes. These are hypertonic (draw normal fluid from the cornea) and can cause further damage and much pain. If a foreign body is present and cannot be flushed out and provided that it is not imbedded in the surface of the eye, one can attempt to lift it out gently with a moist cotton-tipped applicator stick. Never use dry cotton in the eye or any wound. If the eyeball is penetrated, the surface is damaged, or a bluish cast is noted, place the animal in a clean, dust-free stall and call a veterinarian immediately.

With the arrival of the face fly in California, horses there are now commonly affected by a contagious conjunctivitis (inflammation of the lining of the eyelids). This usually occurs late in the summer. This is very similar to "pinkeye" in cattle and in man. Antibiotic eye ointments are frequently effective when they are accompanied by aspirin mixed in with the grain to minimize the pain and reduce local tissue swelling. Very badly inflamed eyes with extensive tissue swelling should receive veterinary attention.

Hematomas

If an animal is kicked or injured so that a blood vessel ruptures under the skin, the swelling that results is called a hematoma (Fig. 124). The most common site for these very large "blood blisters" is on the muscles of the buttock area. This is where most horses kick each other during fights. Initially, the swelling is very flabby and obviously contains free fluid. Always use cold applications at first (e.g., ice packs, 10 to 15 minutes, once or twice daily for 4 days). Never attempt to lance (cut open) or drain a swelling like this for the first 1 to 2 weeks. The injured blood vessels may continue bleeding. After 2 weeks, draining of very large hematomas may be indicated. The removal of the straw-colored fluid causes marked reduction in the size of the swelling. Some increase in size will recur but then the area will get smaller

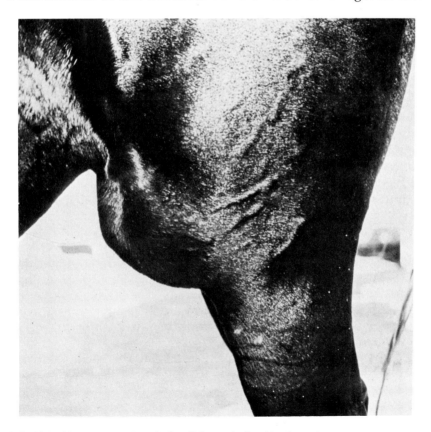

FIG. 124.   Hematoma or "blood blister" from a broken blood vessel.

and begin to become more firm and solid. At this time, the gentle use of heat (e.g., mild liniments or moist heat) can help increase local circulation to speed up the recovery period. The complete disappearance of such swellings most often takes between 4 and 8 weeks. Seldom is there any permanent blemish unless a muscle separation (resulting in an indentation) occurred at the time of the injury.

Saddle Sores

The saddle region of riding horses is frequently affected by local areas of tissue damage. The severity of the problem depends on the amount of damage that has occurred. These "sores" or sore areas may vary from only a small area of swelling and tenderness to more extensive, open, infected wounds.

The most common cause of true saddle sores is a poorly fitted saddle or one not properly padded. Excessive rubbing causes a "galling" or rubbed raw area, which becomes swollen, bare, and very tender. If continued rubbing occurs to the area, an open, infected wound may result.

Treatment

Early cases of local tissue swelling are best treated with cold applications (ice packs), rest, and aspirin (ten 5-grain tablets) twice daily in the grain to reduce tissue swelling. If the area is raw, spraying the area with nitrofurazone (yellow) spray is indicated. This is one case where gentian violet (an astringent) may be helpful, but unfortunately, this medication is too often misused for all types of wounds of the horse.

If an open wound has occurred, it should be treated with an effective, local antibacterial medication such as nitrofurazone powder. An injection of an antibiotic may be needed to treat or prevent an infection.

If it is necessary to ride a horse that has a sore area over the back, this area can often be protected by using first a sponge rubber underpad with a hole cut out of it over the area of the problem. This will usually prevent any further direct pressure on the area. Always use extra saddle pads on any horse with a prominent back bone or withers.

Other causes of local sore swollen areas over the back where the saddle goes are: cattle grubs (ox warbles) and local injury from rolling over on a rock or dirt clod. The treatment of ice packs, aspirin, and perhaps cortisone injections may be needed. Cattle grubs may have to be surgically removed. Much scar tissue under the skin in the saddle area may cause a great deal of irritation and pain to the horse. Surgical removal of this scar tissue may be necessary.

Sprains

A sprain is an injury to a joint caused by wrenching. There is stretching and possible partial rupture of the ligaments and tendons but there is not dislocation or fracture of the bones. If the initial injury were severe, serious damage could have been done. Acute lameness and an enlarged joint with or without swelling extending up above the affected joint may be found. A veterinarian should treat such injuries and the treatment usually consists of the administration of an anti-inflammatory drug and immediate immobilization of the joint. A flexible cast is most often applied. Forced rest in a stall or small paddock is indicated. Less severe sprains can be treated with aspirin twice daily, cold water or ice packs applied once or twice daily, a Vetrap bandage properly padded, and forced rest. Allowing sufficient time for a complete recovery is very important to avoid re-injury and serious damage to the joint.

Fractures

Fractures in the horse still represent a major problem for repair. The major cause of unsuccessful treatment is the difficulty of immobilizing the site of the fracture. This is especially true in heavily muscled areas such as the upper forearm or thigh. Even pinning these fractures and keeping the animal in slings are not guarantees of immobilization. Many horses will continue to fight the sling and the constant movement will not allow the fracture to heal. Fractures in the pastern area also share an extremely poor prognosis. This is true not because this type of fracture is difficult to immobilize; it is not. But as the bones heal, a large calcium deposit invariably results. This produces the same effect as a ring bone—a roughened calcium area on the pastern bones, over which tendons pass, rubbing against this roughened area. Pain and permanent lameness result. If a horse must sustain a broken leg, a fracture of the cannon bone will have the best chances of being repaired successfully. It has no heavy muscles covering it and it can easily be immobilized with a plaster cast. There is a better prognosis for all types of fractures in young horses. Horses with broken legs high in the muscled areas are usually better euthanized, but these and lower fractures should be examined by a veterinarian to instigate possible repair. Any very acute lameness with the animal refusing to bear any weight on the leg should be regarded as a possible fracture. A free, dangling leg is fairly indicative of a fracture. Always try to keep the animal as quiet as possible until the veterinarian can arrive to attend the case. A makeshift splint may be indicated if the doctor is not available in a relatively short time.

First Aid

A simple, but very effective method of temporarily immobilizing a leg fracture is with a pillow. The pillow is applied over the fracture area and is then tightly bound to the leg. Then, use ordinary flannel bandages, applied as tightly as possible. Over that, elastic bandages are applied, again as tightly as possible. If elastic bandages are not available, gauze bandages or ordinary adhesive tape can be used. A broomstick can be incorporated into the bandage to give extra stiffness. This can be used on almost all types of leg fractures. The materials are usually available and the horse does not usually panic. It is safe and can make it possible to move an animal quite a distance for proper medical attention.

Useful Home Remedies

1. Aspirin for any inflammation
2. Antihistamine for any allergic reaction such as bee stings, feed allergies, or early laminitis and congestion in respiratory infections.
3. Hot bran mashes for early mild colics, constipation, and warming up a horse on a cold night.
4. Tincture of green soap with or without a follow-up insecticide bath for many nonspecific skin conditions.
5. Boric acid solution (2 level tablespoons in 8 ounces of water) and antibiotic eye ointments for eye irritation.
6. Noxzema Medicated Cold Cream applied lightly around wounds as a fly repellent.
7. Mud to keep feet soft in summer. Allow water trough to overflow. Also equal parts of lanolin, pine tar, and neat's-foot oil or linseed oil works well as a hoof dressing. The dressing can be made less viscous by adding more of the oil used.
8. Tincture of iodine is very good for thrush. Chlorine bleach and iodine also work but have shorter action. Turpentine is *not* recommended for thrush.

Helpful Nursing Procedures for the Sick Horse

1. Provide a roomy, quiet box stall with good ventilation but without drafts. Avoid extremes in temperature.
2. Keep stall well bedded with clean straw (slightly dampened if dusty). Have clean, fresh water available. Change water bucket frequently.

3. In cold weather or to prevent chilling, a blanket is recommended. Leg bandages are also useful in very cold weather. In the summer, fly sheets add to the patient's comfort.
4. Exercise should be limited. Absolute rest is one of the best treatments for a sick animal, but as the horse begins to feel better, it should receive some exercise as recommended by the attending veterinarian. Overstress and fatigue can worsen the patient's condition.
5. It is important to try to have the animal maintain a good appetite. If a high fever is present, the animal loses interest in eating and constipation may become a problem. A bran mash helps to correct this. Aspirin helps reduce the fever and make the animal feel better. If the horse is not eating well enough to take the aspirin in its feed, the aspirin can be mixed with honey and the mixture can be gobbed into the horse's mouth.

The following can be offered to stimulate its appetite: hot bran mash, steamed oats, chopped apples or carrots, alfalfa meal and molasses, grass, and hay or grain that has been sprinkled with warm molasses or honey and water (half and half). Hand feeding is often helpful.

Suggested Contents for First-Aid Kit

The following are recommended contents for a first-aid kit for horses:
1. Mild surgical soap or L.O.C. and Betadine disinfectant
2. One-pound roll of cotton to be used for cleaning wounds
3. Nitrofurazone powder—puff or spray container for general use on unbandaged wounds
4. Nitrofurazone dressing—salve to apply to a wound under a bandage. Do not apply salve to an open wound
5. Petroleum jelly or hand cream for extra-dry skin areas
6. Caustic powder with copper sulfate to be used only on old wounds beginning to develop proud flesh. Neo-predef powder is best for this
7. Noxzema Medicated Cold Cream or commercial fly repellent to be used around wounds to repel flies
8. Antibiotic eye ointment
9. Kopertox for thrush and minor wounds of hoof coronary band
10. Four sheets of sheet cotton or other padding to be used under bandages
11. Two 1-inch rolls of adhesive or masking tape
12. Two to four (4-inch) Vetrap bandages

CHART IV. ANNUAL ROUTINE HEALTH RECORD

HORSE	Year	Sleeping Sickness	Tetanus Toxoid	Influenza	Rhino-pneumonitis	Other	Teeth

Ⓑ—booster

RECOMMENDED SCHEDULE

Vaccinations   In the spring or as directed by your veterinarian.

Worming   As directed by your veterinarian.

Teeth   Annual exam to determine if floating is needed. Most horses require floating at least once a year; many at only 6-month intervals, start routine teeth examinations from 18 months of age.

Feet   Hooves should be trimmed or reshod at 6- to 8-week intervals. Many horses require monthly attention. The average is 6 weeks.

Sheath   Clean sheath at least every 6 months.

13. One 4-inch roll of Elastron, a rubber elastic tape
14. Mild liniment to be used only when indicated by a veterinarian or bottle of DMSO
15. Small box of 3 × 3-inch sterile gauze pads
16. Pair of curved scissors to clip hair around a wound or to trim ragged wound edges that are *not* to be sutured
17. Twitch—a small twitch can be made of a 14-inch length of dog collar chain attached to a double snap. After applying the twist on the nose, the twitch can be clipped to the halter
18. Chart on proper wound treatment

PART
IV

Appendices

APPENDIX

A

Questions and Answers

The following questions and answers are related to common problems the author observes routinely in his equine veterinary practice.

1. What are the most common errors people make when purchasing a horse?
   Answer: (a) getting a green-broke horse (untrained) for a novice or very young rider, (b) buying a very nervous or otherwise unsuitable horse, (c) not taking enough time to properly select the right horse.

2. What are the most common errors owners make in providing stabling facilities for their horse(s)?
   Answer: (a) barbwire fences, (b) insecure gates, (c) inadequate space, (d) poor bedding in stalls, (e) not having an area in wet weather where horses can get out of the mud, (f) not providing a safe area for the foaling mare.

3. What is one of the most commonly neglected grooming procedures?
   Answer: Cleaning the sheath of geldings or stallions on a routine basis (at least once every 6 months); also frequent routine cleaning of the feet.

4. How often should horses be shod?
   Answer: Most horses should be shod at 6- to 8-week intervals with 6 weeks being the average. Some horses need to be reshod at 4-week intervals, although a few can go as long as 10 weeks between shoeings.

5. If a horse is left barefoot, how often should its hooves be trimmed?

   Answer: At least every 8 weeks. If a horse is being used frequently while being left barefoot, trimming every 4 weeks keeps its hooves from chipping and splitting.

6. Is it a good practice to have a horse's shoes removed for the winter?

   Answer: This is a common practice and is probably good for most horses if they are still trimmed on a regular basis (at least once every 6 to 8 weeks). Horses with very thin walls or other foot problems that require corrective shoes usually must be routinely shod the year around.

7. What is teeth floating?

   Answer: Horses teeth grow throughout their entire lives. Because the back chewing teeth overlap (the uppers to the outside and the lowers to the inside) as they wear, they develop very sharp points and edges that cut into the cheeks and tongue. This makes it painful for the horse to chew well and lowers its ability to utilize food. Also, improperly chewed hay predisposes the horse to impactions (blocked intestines). Floating the teeth is the filing down of these sharp points by a veterinarian.

8. What is the age when horses need to have their teeth floated?

   Answer: Many horses only 18 months old have very sharp dental points and need these filed down to maximize feed utilization and to eliminate the pain caused by these sharp points. The author has observed cheek lacerations from sharp dental points in colts as young as 4 months of age.

9. How often do horses need their teeth floated?

   Answer: It is common for horses to need their teeth floated every 6 months. Some horses may go as long as 2 years before significant points develop and cause mouth injuries. Horses should be checked and have their teeth floated at least annually.

10. What are the most common errors owners make in feeding their horses?

    Answer: (a) not feeding enough according to specific needs, especially in the case of the nursing mare and the growing foal, (b) turning horses out to pasture in the winter with no food supplements, (c) turning old horses "out to pasture" when they most often need extra care and a special diet that is easy to digest, (d) not supplying a vitamin supplement, especially vitamin A, which is almost always deficient in feeds stored 6 months or longer, (e) feeding a diet that has a mineral imbalance (especially Ca:P), which commonly causes sore backs and sore joints.

11. What age should horses first be bred?
    Answer: As a rule, it is best to breed horses that are at least 3 years of age and well developed. Occasionally, 2-year-olds are developed well enough for breeding.

12. What are the most common causes for infertility in the mare?
    Answer: (a) low hormone activity and (b) not breeding at the proper time.

13. Are infections a common cause of infertility in the mare?
    Answer: They are not uncommon and must be treated properly if there is hope of having the mare conceive and deliver a healthy foal. Breeding mares that are in the "foaling heat" (9 days after giving birth to a foal) is very likely to predispose the mare to a uterine infection or is likely to result in an abortion or diseased foal.

14. What is one of the most common causes of infertility in the stallion?
    Answer: Failure to ejaculate. The stallion may cover the mare satisfactorily but fail to ejaculate. If this is recognized and the stallion is immediately allowed to recover the mare, he will most often have a successful ejaculation.

15. Is it common for mares to carry their foals longer than the expected 345 days?
    Answer: Yes. It is not uncommon for a mare to carry a normal, healthy foal for as long as 13 months.

16. How early can a foal be born ahead of the expected 335- to 345-day gestation period and be expected to be normal?
    Answer: Foals born 3 weeks early often show signs of being premature.

17. What are the most common mistakes owners make in regard to the foaling mare?
    Answer: (a) allowing her to foal with other horses, which often attack the newborn foal and (b) not having the mare and foal in an enclosed area with a safe fence that is built very close to the ground; newborn foals often roll under a fence and find themselves with other horses or in dangerous areas.

18. What is the best sign a young foal is sick?

Answer: Its lack of appetite. A young foal normally nurses about every 15 minutes or less; when it is not nursing, the mare's udder usually becomes distended and milk often drips down the mare's legs.

19. Are most illnesses of the newborn serious?
   Answer: Yes. Young foals can die easily and should receive proper veterinary attention if they don't appear to be healthy.

20. Is there any procedure that is helpful in preventing most post-foaling problems and infections in the mare and the foal?
   Answer: Yes. The routine examination by a veterinarian of the mare and foal and the administration of antibiotics and tetanus inoculations to them both within the first 24 to 48 hours after the foal's being born has proven to be effective in preventing approximately 90% of post-foaling problems and infections.

21. How long is it usually necessary to keep a foal separated from its dam while weaning it?
   Answer: Usually about 6 weeks. Only a good, safe fence separating them is necessary for this weaning period.

22. What is the most important disease problem that affects horses the world over?
   Answer: Internal parasites (worms). All horses (probably without exception) have some degree of internal worm infestation. They are exposed to an environment of these parasites from the day they are born and many even before they are born.

23. How many major groups of internal parasites do horses normally have?
   Answer: Most often four: blood worm (strongyles), roundworms (ascrids), pinworms, and bots.

24. Is there one worm medicine that is effective against all the common internal parasites of horses?
   Answer: Yes, Ivermectin, which is also approved for use in pregnant mares.

25. How often should horses be wormed?
   Answer: Four to six times a year, or as directed by your veterinarian.

26. Is it a good policy to alternate worm medicines?
   Answer: This has been true; check with your veterinarian for specific advice.

27. How old should a foal be when it is first wormed?
    Answer: Usually about 8 weeks old, sometimes younger. Iver-
    mectin is not recommended for foals younger than 4
    months.

28. What are the most common external parasites of horses?
    Answer: (a) lice, (b) ticks, and (c) ringworm. These are all
    usually winter problems and can cause severe anemia,
    weight loss, and general debility.

29. What is the best medication to use against these parasites?
    Answer: A specific insecticide bath is most effective. Contact
    a veterinarian for specific recommendations.

30. What is the most common infectious disease of horses?
    Answer: The respiratory infections (colds) are the most com-
    mon. Proper treatment and nursing are important in pre-
    venting prolonged illnesses and complications.

31. What are the most common diseases that horses are routinely
    vaccinated against?
    Answer: Sleeping sickness (Eastern, Western), tetanus, influ-
    enza, and rhinopneumonitis.

32. Which is or are the most important?
    Answer: Tetanus because it is so widespread, but also sleeping
    sickness, especially in areas where they pose serious
    threats. The influenza and rhinopneumonitis vaccines are
    very helpful in preventing these debilitating diseases—es-
    pecially in race and show horses. The rhinopneumonitis
    vaccine can also be helpful in preventing abortions caused
    by this virus. (Note: There is a vaccine for the prevention
    of strangles and it is used on many farms and in stables
    where the disease is a recurrent problem.)

33. What is a health program that is commonly utilized by many
    horse owners with their veterinarian?
    Answer: Many veterinarians utilize and recommend the fol-
    lowing general horse health program:
        a) An effective worming program. Contact your veteri-
    narian for specific recommendations.
        b) Horses are commonly vaccinated for sleeping sickness,
    tetanus, influenza, and rhinopneumonitis (strangles also
    when needed) in the spring, along with the worming.
        c) Dental examinations at least once a year. Horses usually
    need their teeth floated annually and many as often as every
    6 months.

34. What is potentially the most serious disease of horses because it is the most common cause of death in the pleasure horse?
    Answer: Colic. Most all colic cases should receive veterinary attention.

35. What general care procedures can an owner take in preventing this serious problem?
    Answer: (a) worm horses on a routine schedule, (b) have teeth floated regularly, (c) never feed moldy feed (store feed well to prevent its getting wet and thus moldy), (d) avoid accidentally overfeeding of grain (secure grain in locked area).

36. Where is the site of most lamenesses in the horse?
    Answer: The foot. Approximately 80% of all equine lameness originates in the foot. (Note: Shoulder lamenesses are very rare.)

37. What are some of the most common causes of lamenesses in the pleasure horse?
    Answer: (a) stone bruises, (b) nail punctures, (c) sprains, (d) navicular disease.

38. Is navicular disease serious and can it be effectively treated?
    Answer: It is very serious; it progresses from a painful bursitis to a degenerative arthritis and eventually causes permanent lameness unless it is treated. It can be effectively treated. Presently the treatment of choice is surgery—neurectomy (cutting of the nerves). This procedure results in an 80% recovery rate, especially if any extra nerve branches are also removed during the surgery.

39. Is there a general treatment that is helpful for many non-specific skin conditions?
    Answer: Often the bathing of a horse with tincture of green soap helps clear up many skin problems. Many cases are caused by parasites or allergies. It is best to consult a veterinarian for a proper diagnosis and treatment program.

40. What is the most important concept to remember when administering a first-aid treatment in the case of a sprain or swelling?
    Answer: Use cold—not hot! Cold constricts local blood vessels and minimizes swelling. Hot can often make it worse. Ice packs or cold water from a hose is useful. Supportive bandages, well padded, are often very helpful.

41. What is one of the most common mistreatments of deep cuts by owners?

Answer: The application of an astringent drying medication, such as gentian violet or a caustic powder. Such medication kills the top layer of cells in the injured area and such injured tissue will eventually have to slough out to be replaced by new cells. Such treatments most often make suturing of these wounds impossible. If a wound needs sutures (stitches), do not use anything but soap and water to clean it until a veterinarian comes, unless he has prescribed some initial medication.

42. Why should salves not be placed on deep wounds if such wounds are to be left unbandaged?
    Answer: Salves applied to open wounds accumulate dirt and debris and may predispose the wound to infection.

43. Is there any group of drugs that can be applied to wounds that is especially helpful in preventing infections in the wounds of horses?
    Answer: Yes, the nitrofurazones. Contact a veterinarian for specific recommendations.

44. Should all wounds of horses be considered potential sources of tetanus?
    Answer: Yes. Tetanus is a universal problem and because horses and humans are so highly susceptible, we should keep both of our immunities up. Many cases of tetanus in the horse occur without the owner recognizing a previous wound, so prevention is definitely best.

45. What procedures can be taken to minimize the chances of a wound developing proud flesh in wounds low in the legs?
    Answer: Minimize its exposure to moisture and debris. Only wash the wound thoroughly on the first treatment. Then try not to apply any water or other liquid to it if possible in future treatments. Allow the wound to heal in to "skin level," then neomycin-cortisone or caustic powder should be applied when left as an open wound. Contact a veterinarian for a specific course of treatment.

46. What is one of the most serious unsoundnesses that affects the suitability of an animal for use as a pleasure horse?
    Answer: Bad temperament. No matter how beautiful, physically sound, or cheap a horse is, if it has a bad temperament, it can be dangerous to have and certainly is no fun to own.

B

Signs and Symptoms

ABNORMAL BEHAVIOR. Horses can demonstrate unusual behavior from a number of different causes. Excessive nervousness can often be from a greater need for vitamin B. Central nervous system problems most often result from direct injury, migrating parasites, or viral infection such as sleeping sickness. Abdominal pain causes rolling, pawing, and getting up and down, which are symptoms of colic.

ABORTION. Almost invariably, mares carrying twins will abort them, usually between the fifth and seventh months. Occasionally, they will be carried full-term, but will be born dead. Rarely do twins live. Direct injury seldom causes an abortion. Phosphorus deficiency can be a cause, as can the rhinopneumonitis virus, uterine infections, and hormonal problems.

CONSTIPATION. This is not an uncommon problem in the aged horse with dental problems and with a less-resilient intestinal tract. Dental problems, intestinal parasites, and very coarse hays or very finely crushed grains can predispose horses to impactions.

COUGHING. Most coughs result from respiratory infections. In young horses, they are commonly caused by migrating parasites. Dusty feeds or allergies are also common causes. Coughs that are improperly treated, or not treated at all, can result in chronic bronchitis or emphysema.

DIARRHEA. This is a common problem in 9-day-old foals, apparently caused by the mare's heat cycle affecting the milk. Vitamin A deficiency, blood worms, and lice can be causes as well as mouldy feeds and certain micro-organisms.

DROOPY EARS most often result from ear ticks, but unusual ear carriage and flicking of the ears can be caused by very small flies that bite and suck blood from inside the lining of the ears.

DRY FEET. Horses being kept in areas during the summer that do not allow for any exposure to moisture can result in dry feet. Vitamin A deficiency is also a common cause. Allowing the water trough to overflow or giving the animal a vitamin A supplement that contains fatty acids designed to improve hair coat are very helpful. Many commercial hoof dressings are also useful, but mud is hard to beat for this purpose.

EXCESSIVE SALIVATION is most often caused by feeding the horse very coarse hay with foxtails or bearded barley. Occasionally, a small stick or piece of very coarse stalk of hay gets jammed between the upper arcade of the teeth across the palate, causing much salivation and making it almost impossible for the horse to chew and swallow. Bad teeth and other causes are not uncommon.

HEAD TOSSING with the bit is usually due to pain caused by the bit hitting against wolf teeth. Ear ticks can be another cause.

ITCHING. Lice are the most common cause of skin irritation to horses. Improperly diluted insecticides can also be a common problem, as can other skin problems.

LACK OF SWEATING is most often a specific symptom of heat-stroke. Patchy sweating is frequently observed in horses near exhaustion.

LIMPING is a symptom of lameness that can be best observed at the trot. It can result from many causes. Hoof stone bruises and puncture wounds are among the most common causes in the pleasure horse.

MANURE EATING, also called "pica," is routine among young foals as they explore their new surroundings. It may also be the result of mineral or feed deficiencies.

NASAL DISCHARGES are most often the result of upper respiratory tract infections. Occasionally, a horse has a frothy, green nasal discharge that is a symptom of vomiting. Horses can vomit, contrary to many beliefs, but the vomitus is directed up through the nostrils because horses have very long, soft palates. Bot irritation in the stomach can cause a horse to vomit.

NERVOUSNESS can just be part of the basic temperament of a

particular horse, but it may also result from an animal having a higher vitamin B complex requirement.

PEELING OF THE SKIN ON THE NOSE, which is usually observed in horses with white muzzles out on pasture in the early spring, results from certain plants in the pasture causing the horses to become sensitive to sunlight (solar dermatitis).

POINTING is when a horse at rest places one front foot out in front of the other. This is a sign that the foot is in pain.

POOR STAMINA can result from many causes such as poor or inadequate nutrition, parasitism, or disease.

POT BELLY is a common symptom of young horses heavily parasitized with ascrids. A low-protein diet of large quantities of poor-quality hay also causes "hay bellies."

RUNNY EYES are commonly caused by a vitamin A deficiency. Horses with no pigmentation around the eyes are often sensitive to sunlight (white horses, bald-faced horses, many Appaloosas) and can be helped by using a black dye or pigment around the eyes during the summer months. Face flies can be a problem, and eye injuries, foreign bodies, such as foxtails, or occasionally a partially blocked nasolacrymal duct can be causes. Secondary discharge from the eyes is not uncommon with respiratory infections.

SKIN BUMPS are most often due to feed allergies or insect bites, especially ticks, but can also be a reaction to insecticides.

SHIVERING most often results from the horse being chilled in wet, cold weather but may be secondary to shock or pain.

SLOW EATING, DIFFICULT CHEWING, AND SWALLOWING most often result from the same causes as those of excessive salivation. Star thistle poisoning can be a specific cause.

STIFFNESS in both front feet is most often caused by laminitis or navicular disease, but sore backs and "tying up" can result in overall stiffness.

STOCKING UP OF THE HIND LEGS can result from low blood protein from internal parasites, plus a lack of exercise. The swelling up of all four legs can result from a general allergic reaction, purpura hemorrhagica, or equine infectious anemia.

SWEATING is normal to cool the body but excessive sweating can be caused by poor conditioning of a horse, too much molasses in the diet, overall insufficient diet, anemia from parasitism, or a combination of these.

SWELLING OF THE CHEST can be caused by direct injury from a kick, causing a hematoma. Constant rubbing against the edge of a manger can cause a seroma (an accumulation of serum under the skin). The swelling may be an abscess.

SWELLING ALONG THE LOWER BELLY WALL (an "abdominal plaque") is a common occurrence in a mare very late in pregnancy and is associated with her "making bag." It is not a serious problem and can be minimized by giving her aspirin in her grain for 4 or 5 days. It always goes away shortly after the foal is born. In California, abscesses frequently occur in this area in late summer.

SWELLING OF THE SHEATH is most commonly caused by the horse standing around in the winter with minimal exercise (this could be secondary to low-blood protein), a dirty sheath, vetch hay allergy, or chronic abscesses.

SIGNS OF FOALING NEAR. The most helpful signs are "waxing over" and the relaxation of the vulva.

SWOLLEN UDDER is most often a symptom of pregnancy but may result from vetch hay allergy or abscesses. Occasionally mastitis, an infection of the mammary gland, can be the cause.

TAIL RUBBING is usually a symptom of a dirty sheath or pinworms. Lice or a local skin irritation can be the cause but not nearly as often as the above.

TENDERNESS OVER THE BACK can be caused by a number of factors but nutrition seems to be the basic, underlying cause, especially the calcium-phosphorus ratio and vitamin B needs.

THIRD EYELIDS UP is observed when the eyes appear to have a membrane covering the inner one-third of both eyes. This is a diagnostic sign of tetanus.

WOOD CHEWING is a common activity of many horses and may be the result of boredom (often developing into a habit), possible mineral deficiency, lack of bulk in the diet, mouth irritation from the migration of bot larvae, or one or more of these conditions in combination.

BIBLIOGRAPHY

Abrams, J.T.: Animal Nutrition and Veterinary Dietetics. Baltimore, Williams & Wilkins, 1962.

Bailey, H.: Vitamin E—Your Key to a Healthy Heart. New York, ARCO, 1970.

Coffman, J.R.: Equine Clinical Chemistry and Pathophysiology. Santa Barbara, Veterinary Medicine Publishing Company, 1982.

Cunha, T.J.: Suggested nutrient levels for horses. Feedstuffs. August 20, 1960:62.

Department of the Army: Veterinary Technicians. Technical Manual TM8-450. Washington, D.C., U.S. Printing Office, 1951.

Eisenmenger, E., and Zetner, K.: Veterinary Dentistry. Philadelphia, Lea & Febiger, 1985.

Ensminger, M.E.: Horses and Horsemanship. Danville, Illinois, Interstate Printers and Publishers, 1977.

Evans, J.W.: Horses. San Francisco, W.H. Freeman, 1977.

Harper, F.: Top Form Book of Horse Care. New York, Popular Library, 1966.

Henricson, B.: Oxytetracycline supplement of rations of colts. Vet. Rec. 72(26):515, 1960.

Hintz, H.F., et al.: Energy requirements of light horses for various activities. J. Animal Science, 32:100, 1971.

Johnson, R.: Training Work Schedules. Personal Communication, 1971 and 1984.

Johnston, R.H. et al.: Mare's milk composition as related to foal heat scours. J. Animal Science, 31:549, 1971.

Jones, W.E.: Genetics and Horse Breeding. Philadelphia, Lea & Febiger, 1982.

Kays, J.M.: The Horse. New York, ARCO, 1977.

Lewis, L.D.: Feeding and Care of the Horse. Philadelphia, Lea & Febiger, 1982.

Mannsmann, R.A., and McAllister, S. (eds.): Equine Medicine and Surgery. 3rd Ed. American Veterinary Publications, 1982.

Maynard, L.A., et al.: Animal Nutrition. 7th Ed. New York, McGraw-Hill, 1979.

McGee, W.R.: Veterinary Notebook. Lexington, The Blood Horse, 1958.

Morrison, F.B.: Feeds and Feeding. Ithaca, Morrison Publishing Company, 1957.

National Research Council: Recommended Nutrients Allowances for Horses. Washington, D.C., National Academy of Science, 1978.

Roberts, J.: Veterinary Obstetrics and Genital Diseases. Ithaca, Published by the author, 1971.

Robinson, N.E.: Current Therapy in Equine Medicine. Philadelphia, W.B. Saunders, 1983.

Schryver, H.F., et al.: Calcium: Phosphorous Interrelationships in Horse Nutrition. Ithaca, Second Equine Nutrition Research Symposium, 1970.

Siegmund, O.H. (Ed): The Merck Veterinary Manual. 5th Ed. Rahway, New Jersey, Merck & Co., 1979.

Soulsby, E.J.L.: Helminths, Arthropods, and Protozoa of Domesticated Animals. 7th Ed. Philadelphia, Lea & Febiger, 1982.

Stashak, T.S.: Adams' Lameness in Horses. 4th Ed. Philadelphia, Lea & Febiger, in preparation.

INDEX

Feet, care of, 74–78
  structure, 76
Fence chewing, 193
Fences, 24, 257
Fever, 209, 219, 237
Firing, 52, 261
First aid kit, 275–276
Fistulous withers, 54
"Fit" animals, 114
  "flagging" of tail, 152
Flies, control of, 207–208
Floating of teeth, 82–83
Foaling, eminent signs of, 156–157
  preparations for, 157–159
  times for assistance, 160–165
Foals, care of newborn, 167–170
  diseases, 170–175
  feeding, 120
  orphan, 123
  turning out, 177–178
Founder. *See* Laminitis
Fractures, 273–274
  sesamoid, 47
Frog (of foot), pressure, 77–78

Galvayne's groove, 39–40
Gelding (castration), 31
Gestation, 140
Grain requirements, 113–118
Granulation tissue, 269
Grass, for feed, 93
"Grass founder," 127, 231
"Graveled," 48
Grooming, 66–69
Grubs, cattle, 202–203

Habronema (stomach worms), 195–196
Hack work, 114
Hand breeding procedure, 145
Handling the horse, 27–28
"Hard keepers," 126
Hay fever, 58
Head shy, 201
Head tossing, 28, 65, 80
Health, good, signs of, 183–184
Heart rate, 184
Heat periods, 139
Heatstroke, 237
Heaveline, 58
Heaves, 58
Heel fly, 202
Hematomas, 271–272
Hernia, 59
Hiplock, 165
History of the horse, 3–4
Hock, capped, 64
Home remedies, 274
Hoof puncture wounds, 46–48

Hooves, dry, 75
  grooving of, 232
Horses, industry in U.S. today, 4–5
  parts of, 2
  populations in U.S., 5
  signs of good health, 183–184
Hygiene, breeding, 142–143
Hypothyroidism, 127, 148

Impaction, 227
  meconium, 170
Infantile uterus, 151
Infertility, 146–153
  mare, 146–147
  stallion, 152–153
Inflammation, 258–261
Influenza, equine, 212–213
Injuries, common causes of, 257
  treatment of, 259–277
Insect bites, 140, 239
Insurance, health, 33
  surgical, 33
Intestinal obstruction, 191
Intra-abdominal bleeding, 166
Ivermectin, 198

"Joint ill," 172
Jumping, 115

Kicking, 22, 65
"Knock kneed," 175

Lacerations, 23, 262, 265
Lameness, 44–52, 189
  common causes of, 286
Laminitis, 24, 46, 54–55, 231–232
  chronic, 79–80
Legs, crooked, in foals, 175–176
  swollen ("stocked up"), 215, 225
Lice, 199–201, 238–239
Life expectancy, 31
Limping, 45–46
Liniments, 261
Linseed meal, 98
L.O.C., 70, 72, 263, 275
Lockjaw (tetanus), 216–218
Lumbar myositis (sore back), 60, 232, 235
Lung congestion, 209

Mane pulling, 69
Manure, disposal of, 207
Mare(s), breeding physiology of, 139
  foaling, care of, 154–166
  nursing, drying up, 180
  feeding program for, 126